WORLD ON EDGE

WILLIAM SARGENT

Table of Contents

Acknowledgements

Prologue
Verkhoyansk											10

Durban

Chapter 1
"It Was a Dark and Stormy Night"							14

Chapter 2
Living on the Edge: Floods								16

Chapter 3
Living on the Edge: Fire								20

Chapter 4
"We Have Met the Enemy and He is us"						22

Chapter 5
The Tipping Point									26

Chapter 6
The First Tesla System in Ipswich;							28

Chapter 7
Dragonflies;The Calm After the Storm						30

Chapter 8
Ida, Katrina and Infrastructure							34

Chapter 9
Afghanistan										36

Chapter 10
Cruising the Parker River Wildlife Refuge						38

Chapter 11
Hurricane Larry; One Strange Bird							40

Chapter 12
A Short Story About a Long Snake							42

Chapter 13
Guy Walks Into a Bar... Plankton, Mammoth and Otters				44

Chapter 14
The Crack in Cumbre Vieja								48

Chapter 15
Horseshoe Crabs and Covid-19							52

Chapter 16
"Regular Gas, $3.42"   56

Chapter 17
Sequestering Carbon, Nature's Way   58

Chapter 18
Sequestering Carbon, The Industrial Way   62

Chapter 19
Methane; Glasgow's Key to Success?   64

Chapter 20
Think Global, Act Local   66

Chapter 21
Sharks and Seals; Worms and Coronaviruses   70

Chapter 22
Shark Attack!   72

Chapter 23
Sequestering Carbon; One Whale at a Time?   74

Chapter 24
Building Our Way out of the Environmental Crisis; Will it work?   76

Chapter 25
The Healing   78

Chapter 26
Resource Wars; Cobalt   80

Chapter 27
The Glasgow Fiasco   82

Chapter 28
Oysters; Ocean Acidification Threatens One of our Proudest Industries. 84

Chapter 29
"Like a Big Bomb"   88

Chapter 30
Fusion; Energy's New Hope?   92

Chapter 31
The Pipeline   94

Chapter 32
Manganese Nodules; Cobalt for the Future?   96

Chapter 33
The Island   100

Chapter 34
The Emergency!   102

Chapter 35
Aftermath   106

Chapter 36
Could Seals Harbor the Next Pandemic?   108

Chapter 37
"Do you have a problem with that … Deer?"*Covid-19 and Climate Change*   112

Chapter 38
The End of Barrier Beaches   114

Chapter 39
The E. O. Wilson East Coast Wildlife Corridor   118

Chapter 40
The Invasion   120

Chapter 41
Weapons the World Thought Would Never be Used   124

Chapter 42
The Budapest Memorandum   126

Chapter 43
A Turning Point?   128

Chapter 44

The Exposure   130

Sources   136

ACKNOWLEDGEMENTS

Most of the people who helped make this book happen are mentioned in the text. But I would like to send a special shout out to Becky Coburn who did her usual wonderful job editing the book and shepherding it through the publishing process. Jill Buchanan did her usual wonderful job designing our cover.

I would also like to thank John Muldoon who published many of the chapters in this book in my weekly column in the Ipswich Local News. Dan Graovac provided some of the beautiful natural history photos featured in the book.

This book was made possible with grants from the Quebec Labrador Foundation, The Sounds Conservancy and Andy Griffith with Plum Island Outdoors who sponsored many of our regular natural history walks.

PROLOGUE
Verkhoyansk
June 20, 2021

The first thing you notice when you drive into Verkhoyansk Siberia are two fifteen-foot mammoth tusks looming up ahead in your headlights.

The statue commemorates that this Ostrog founded by Cossacks once held the record for the coldest temperature in the Northern Hemisphere. It was minus 38 degrees Centigrade — minus 90 degrees Fahrenheit.

But on June 20th 2021, the temperature hit 100.4 degrees Fahrenheit — a 190-degree temperature range in a single location.

The tusks come from the banks of the Yana River just outside of Verkhoyansk. The climate is now so mild in Siberia that the permafrost is melting, so the frozen carcasses of mammoths erode out of the banks of the river.

Looters use pumps to melt the permafrost with bursts of hot water. Six had to be airlifted off Bolshoy Lyakhovsky Island in October. They ran out of supplies and were starving. The situation was getting to be as out of control as Kaliningrad's illegal trade in fossil filled amber.

But Verkhoyanskians aren't very concerned about what climate change will do to their agriculture. In fact they look forward to growing Siberian wheat and shipping it across the ice-free Arctic to Asia.

It sounds almost as good as when Comrade Lysenko said you could train summer wheat to grow in Siberia. His anti-evolutionary ideology set back Soviet science for decades.

Verkhoyanskians are pleased that Russian icebreakers can now break through the thin summer ice. It used to be 10 meters thick, now it is thin and riddled with holes which Siberians call "polynya".

Durban: January 1, 2022

Durban South Africa sits on the Indian Ocean, 9,517 miles to the south of Siberia. It's in the humid province of KwaZulu-Natal, which received its Portuguese name from Vasco de Gama, who explored this coast while looking for a southern route to Asia. Since it was Christmas he gave the area the Portuguese name "Natal". Locals just call their city "Durbs."

Its population is a cosmopolitan mix of Zulu, British and Indian decent. Mahatma Gandhi practiced law here as a young man.

Durban is also home to Dr. Richard Lessells, who discovered that the omicron variant probably came from an unfortunate young woman who had both HIV and Covid-19.

Someone had botched her treatment so she had not been given HIV anti-virals. This had given her load of Covid viruses over a month to mutate, over a month to become a hundred times more contagious but several times less deadly, a most efficient, almost perfect parasite.

Unknowingly her doctors had been doing Gain of Function Research on a human being instead of a lab animal and it had led to the Omicron variant that was sweeping around the globe. She would go down with Typhoid Mary, the cook who infected thousands and Gaetan Dugas, the Quebecois flight attendant known for infecting hs casual sex partners with HIV, then telling them he had given them "gay cancer".

The doctor who failed to follow protocol and give the young woman anti-virals should join the Chinese Gain of Function researcher, who purportedly became Patient Zero after the ferret he was injecting with Covid sneezed, wiggled or bit him on the thumb, making him Covid's Patient Zero.

So as the third year of Covid began, scientists were transfixed with three locations on opposites antipodes of our planet. The Arctic Circle, where it had soared over 100 degrees; Washington, where Joe Manchin, a single senator, was topedoeing America's attempt to stop global warming, and South Africa, where a negligent doctor had probably launched Covid-19 on its new fast moving trajectory.

So far Covid had killed more people than almost all the wars in history, and the global economy was teetering on the edge. Population growth was the lowest it had ever been since the founding of the United States. People were traveling less, walking more, eating better, buying fewer consumables, going outside, even being more spiritual.

Had nature stepped in to solve the environmental crisis on her own? We will have to revisit the momentous year 2021 to see.

CHAPTER 1
"It Was a Dark and Stormy Night"
Lytton, British Columbia
June 29, 2021

Lytton, British Columbia is a bucolic little village that spans the confluence of the Fraser and Thompson Rivers. Most of its 250 inhabitants are indigenous Canadians who have lived on this land for over 10,000 years.

The rest are descendants of non-indigenous settlers who came during the Fraser Canyon Gold Rush in 1858. The inhabitants hunt, fish, work in the forestry industry and run raft trips.

The village was named for the 19th century writer Lord Bulwer-Lytton who opened his book *Paul Clifford* with the immortal line, "It was a dark and stormy night".

Unfortunately it was not dark and stormy on June 29, 2021.

Instead temperatures rose to a thermometer popping 121 degrees farenheit. It was the highest temperature ever recorded this far north, the highest recorded in the United States and Canada except for America's 4 desert states, and it was higher than any temperatures ever reached in either Europe or South America. It had culminated the world's hottest June ever recorded in human history.

The very next day a wildfire destroyed 90% of the village, which was trapped under a dome of high-pressure air that had caused triple digit heat waves in cities like Portland and Seattle and caused 500 deaths in Canada alone.

The hellish heat had caused droughts, shriveled crops, threatened water supplies and was leading up to what looked like the worst wildfire season in memory.

But the high temperatures were not restricted to North America. Europe had suffered its second warmest June on record and temperatures had also been above average in Africa, the Middle East and China.

And unfortunately the extreme temperatures were expected to last well into September. All we could do was pray for a succession of dark and stormy nights.

Chapter 2
Living on the Edge: Floods
Ipswich, Massachusetts
July 18, 2021

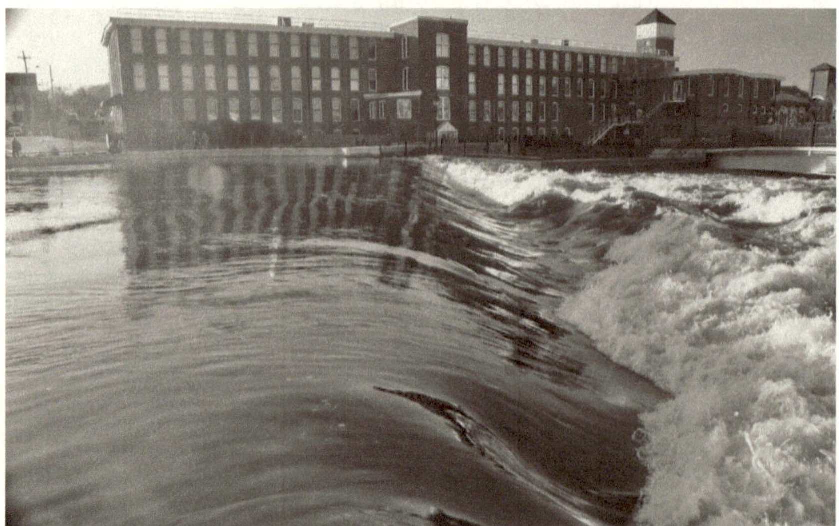

Floods

It was early dawn when I woke to the sharp sound of rain pelting my window and cascading down the sides of our house. My thoughts raced to my car. Its sunroof had developed a leak that had soaked the back seat floor.

I had parked on a steep hill so the water could drain out from under the car. As I approached I could hear water rushing under a manhole as it whooshed down the hill toward the waiting Atlantic. I knew if I didn't get my car fixed soon, I would end up with fetid water, mold, and electrical problems. I would probably have to sell my much beloved new car.

But I also knew was lucky. Over 300 people had just died and thousands more were missing from floods in West Germany. In China, floods had misplaced 1.2 million people, and trapped hundreds more in subways where at least 25 had drowned in neck deep water.

On television, I watched SUVs jauntily bobbing up and down in the swollen Rhine River on their way to the Netherlands. There, the water was spreading out over the land and gurgling into underground reservoirs. Dutch engineers had moved the farmhouses off the fields and placed them on specially designed high hills and diverted floodwaters into reservoirs they built under tennis courts and parking lots.

After the floods passed, the farmland and cityscapes would dry out and return to normal. It was all part of what the Dutch call *Leben mit dem Wasser*, a policy started after a severe storm where floods drowned 1,800 people storm in 1953.

We have yet to learn such valuable lessons. The fresh water rushing off my glacial drumlin was flowing directly into Plum Island Sound along with runoff, leached sewage and lawn fertilizer.

There, the fresh water was triggering red tide organisms to bloom in deadly abundance. Their cysts had spent the last two years sequestered in the marsh waiting for enough rainwater to release them from their Snow White-like suspended animation. Clam beds had already been closed from Maine to Rhode Island.

The fresh water would allow the red tide organisms to expand their range. Previously such dinoflagellates had only existed north of Cape Cod. But in 1972, heavy rains from tropical storm Carrie had pushed the organisms around the tip of Cape Cod, where they encysted in the brackish mud of the southerly saltwater ponds.

Red tide organisms had also been implicated in James Bond style political assassinations. In 1978, a Bulgarian dissident was boarding a bus in London when he had been jostled by a fellow passenger whose umbrella had jabbed him in the leg. Turns out the umbrella had been specially designed to inject a steel ball filled with paralytic shellfish poison from these same red tide organisms. Hence we get the expression *Bulgarian umbrella* which you definitely don't want to buy, online or off.

While combined sewage outfalls and lawn fertilizer runoff were exacerbating the problem in the north, in Florida a phosphate plant dam had broken and red tide blooms were killing thousands of manatees and dolphins.

Of course that was not the full extent of Florida's water damage. A few weeks before the surfside Condominium had collapsed due to salt water weakening the Condo's cement foundation, a problem also encountered in seaside nuclear power plants.

When he visited the site, President Biden suggested that the saltwater intrusion had been caused by sea level rise. A year before such a suggestion would have been met with screams of denial, but it was getting harder and harder to deny climate change, when the heat domes, humidity, jet stream fluctuations and floods that were on the news every night.

When climate scientists studied climate change forty years ago they debated whether we were going to have a Greenhouse world or an Icehouse world. But several of the most prescient researchers predicted that the jet stream would start to fluctuate wildly north and south creating what they called a Madhouse world. Today it is clear we are right smack dab in the middle of that runaway world.

CHAPTER 3
Living on the Edge: Fire
July 20, 2021

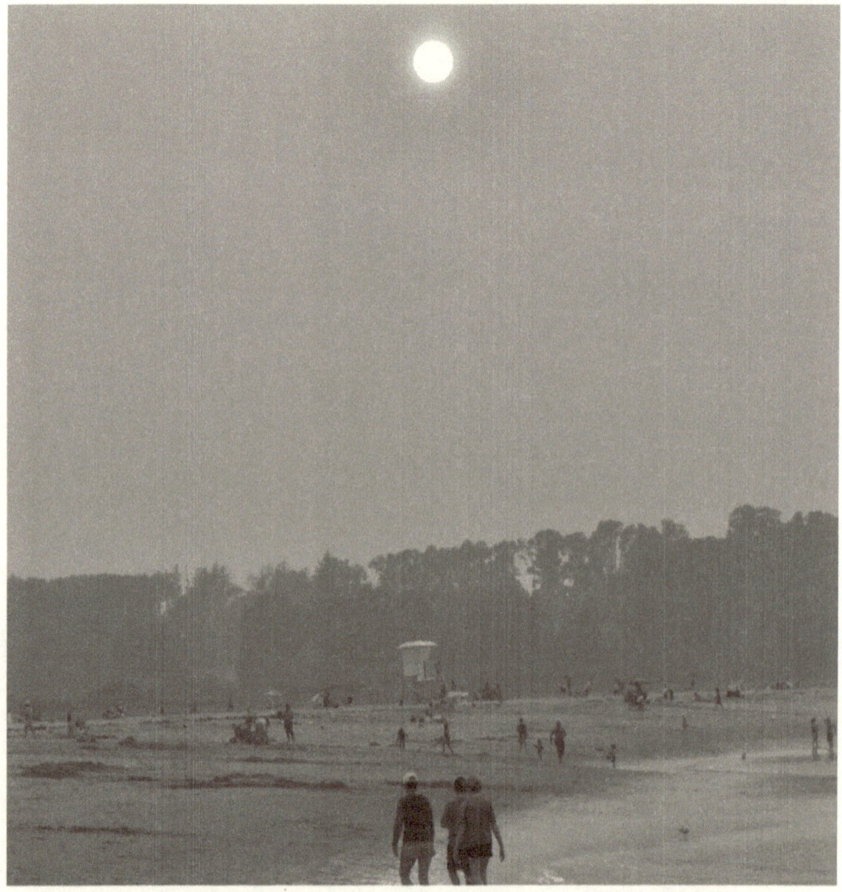

Smoke from Oregon fires cut through the sun on Crane's Beach

It was difficult to breath on July 20. Delta variants were on the rise and the sun skulked behind a pallid blanket of heavy, hot air. It was air that brought back visceral memories of when humanity thought such diseases were caused by bad air from which we get the term *malaria*. But this bad air was caused by something quite different.

The Ipswich Marsh lay behind a sickly bank of fog, haze and smoke, smoke which came from Oregon's Bootleg fire 3,000 miles away. It is just one of 85 fires that were consuming 1.5 million acres of forests on the West Coast.

Heat from the Bootleg fire had created towering clouds of smoke and moisture that boiled up thousands of feet to where airliners would have flown if they had not been diverted because of high winds and lightning generated by Bootleg's fire tornadoes.

Normally the weather determines what a fire will do, but the Bootleg the fire was determining what the weather would do.

The firestorms' erratic behavior was defeating efforts to contain them. They swirled, leapt and jumped over firebreaks, leapfrogging through the canopy igniting distant new spot fires, and creating towering fire tornadoes with 140 mile per hour winds. Firefighters retreated, leaving dead wildlife and scorched earth in the wake of the ever-widening conflagration.

They watched as pyrocumulus clouds rose 30,000 feet in the air then collapsed at night making the air plunge back to the earth where it exploded outwards in strong ember filled gusts that spread the fire in all directions. It was like battling a malevolent, sentient creature.

The week before, the fire had built a 45,000-foot high thunderhead bristling with deadly flashes of lightning. It had created its own rainstorms, but rather than dampening the fires the rain had created more fire, spreading downdrafts by cooling the air closest to the earth. The firemen saved a lone bear cub abandoned in a smoldering tree but paid little heed to cattle roaming freely through the fire-charred ruins.

In less than a month the fires had erased all the carbon dioxide reductions achieved during the last year's pandemic. It was clear that this was going to be the West's worst year for forest fires, and the season had barely begun.

CHAPTER 4
"We Have Met the Enemy and He is us"
Population
July 27, 2021

On July 27, 2021 I drove to nearby Plum Island. It had been ravaged by all four horsemen of the environmental apocalypse.

On land, erosion had unearthed the ruins of a Federal radio facility that used to communicate with Coast Guard cutters from Maine to Florida. At sea, the Merrimack River and the Atlantic Ocean were a sickly muddy brown from sewage that had closed beaches for swimming and red tide organisms that had closed clamflats for shellfishing.

The night before, a storm had washed a heroin needle down the Merrimack from an upstream encampment of drug addicts. Now it lay tangled in the wrackline.

Even the air itself was polluted with the deep gray pallor of smoke from the West Coast fires and masked people were wandering along the shore like desultory zombies. It felt like we were truly living on a dying planet.

But there is one more horseman of this environmental apocalypse, and it is us. The earth's human population has tripled since 1950. Our planet has too many people driving too many cars and having too many children. It is what we like to do.

But a recent Columbia University study found that every year, three Americans release enough carbon to kill a person from heat stroke. It takes about 300 Nigerians to cause the same damage.

When this kind of population explosion occurs in other species, nature takes over and thins the population through predators, plagues, famine or war; the four horsemen again.

When a population of lemmings explodes, the rodents consume all the available lichen and swim out into the Arctic and drown, not so much to commit suicide but in search of more food. When locust populations explode, they are infected by viruses that kill them from within.

When a population of monkeys becomes so large they run out of food, they wage wars on neighboring troops to take over their resources. Or political tensions among dominant males within the troop cause it to split apart and form two groups, one that stays, while the other on to new resource rich areas.

So where to we stand today? So far predators don't seem to be much of a problem. Lions, tigers, bears, sharks and crocodiles only account for a few thousand human deaths every year, and thanks to Sigourney Weaver we seem relatively safe from predatory aliens.

But Covid-19 is the canary in the coalmine that just killed an estimated 10 million humans, more than in all but our most deadly wars. It reduced our average lifespan by several years, but has it thinned our ranks enough to stop our environmental apocalypse?

That depends. Many people expected a baby boom from lockdown boredom. That had happened during blackouts, but it didn't happen this time. Instead, couples made the decision not to have babies when hospitals were backed up with Covid cases and the future was so uncertain.

The same thing happened after the Spanish flu in 1918. That plus World War I killed so many young people in their twenties and thirties, there was a baby bust ,but birth rates recovered. That didn't happen after the 2008 recession, birth rates never went back to their former levels.

So while the four traditional horsemen are clearly not controlling the human population, carbon, Covid-19 and people themselves may do the same thing that happened in 1918 and 2008.

The human population is expected to reach 11 billion in 2100. But our rate of increase had already dropped from 2.2 percent to 1.05 percent. We just lost another 10 million humans to Covid and 8 million to carbon. People have seen and now know the risks and costs of raising children in such an uncertain world. And if we continue to educate and empower women and lower infant mortality there may be a path toward lower population growth.

The World Health Organization has called climate change the greatest threat to human health, and that a runaway hot-earth scenario could lead to a human population collapse. But perhaps plain old common sense, and our Covid induced wakeup call may just lead us to a more sustainable future.

For if we don't control our human population, heat, fires, floods and recurring pandemics will step in and do it for us.

CHAPTER 5
The Tipping Point
August 3, 2021

In early August I awoke to the sharp cries of an osprey circling against another rain- filled sky. It was like someone had flipped a switch, after the earliest heat wave ever in June, it had been New England's rainiest July on record.

Fledgling terns lined up along the shore of Crane's Beach, waiting for their parents to bring them sand launce so slender the three inch morsels slid down their throats like pieces of thin spaghetti.

Offshore, humpback and minke whales, tuna and Great White Shark were feeding on the unusual abundance of menhaden this far north.

Something strange had happened this summer and the answer was lurking in the nearby Gulf Stream and a blob of persistently cold water caused by meltwater flowing off Greenland.

Normally the Gulf Stream carries salty warm water north from the tropics. There it cools, becomes denser and sinks to the ocean floor and flows south again to the tropics. While we like to think of the Gulf Stream driving this system, it is really the sinking of the cold dense water that pulls the Gulf Stream north, like a conveyor belt.

But global warming has started to make the Gulf Stream waters less dense and that plus fresh water flowing off Greenland, have worked in tandem to slow down the Gulf Steam. This is causing cooler weather and floods in Europe, droughts in the mid-West and our unusual but welcome rainy summer that has saved us from our profligate use of rain to overwater our lawns.

But the Gulf Stream won't let us off scot-free. It is already causing favorite seafood species like lobster to move north and northern shorebirds are unable to find enough fatty baitfish to feed their offspring successfully.

As the Gulf Stream slows it will also slacken and pile up against the East Coast. This will raise the already rising tides and seas. We can expect to see these effects in the stronger more frequent hurricanes of late summer and the Northeasters of the coming falls, winters and springs.

CHAPTER 6
The First Tesla System in Ipswich;
A Glimpse of the Future
August 6, 2021

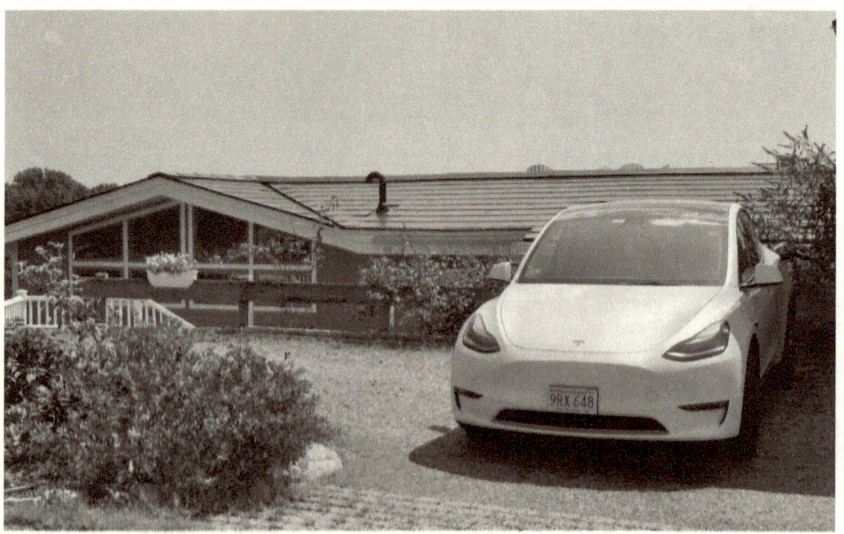

Tesla

On August 6 I caught a glimpse of the future. The neat white lines of a Tesla sat in front of the elegant black glass shingles of a low ranch style house perched below the brow of the hill below. The bright faces of daisies nodded in the breeze. It looked so much like an ad for South California Living; I half expected to see surf roll in from the Pacific.

But I was standing on a glacial drumlin overlooking a New England marsh. The setting sun was shining off the numinous white wings of Great Egrets as they side slipped and braked on their steep descent to the rookery, below.

The daisies nodded beside a sleek black cable charging the Tesla, on its rear window a sticker announced that the owner of the car had been an Audubon member in good standing for the past 25 years. I decided to knock.

Dr. Brown showed me an app on her phone that indicated that at the moment about a third of the electricity being generated by the roof's shingles was being used to charge her car, a third was cooling the house and a third was being returned to the Ipswich electrical supply.

This was the first fully integrated Tesla system in our small town and others in the state were returning more electricity to the grid than all the nuclear power plants in New England.

It all came about when Dr. Brown saw her first Tesla speeding by on the highway. She had to push her Prius to get close enough to see the unassuming T that was the only insignia that heralded the other car as a Tesla. From that moment on the neurologist saw her path to helping protect the environment.

But it was a long process. When she moved from Little Neck to Great Neck she bought a ranch style Acorn house because it perched on the woodsy face of the drumlin overlooking the Ipswich River marsh.

The house had one of the best views on the North Shore but she soon discovered the roof of the house didn't have any studs to hold down traditional solar panels in the high winds and spectacular storms that were also part of living on the Neck.

But when Tesla started producing its elegant black glass shingles in 2015, she knew she had her answer. All she needed was one of the large distinctive batteries that looked a giant Apple I-phone, one suspects by intention.

Dr. Brown knows that she will probably not make back her investment in her lifetime but she is content to know that she is helping herself, her town and the environment, all while helping to bring down the price of future installations.

Chapter 7
Dragonflies; The Calm After the Storm
Ipswich, Massachusetts
August 24, 2021

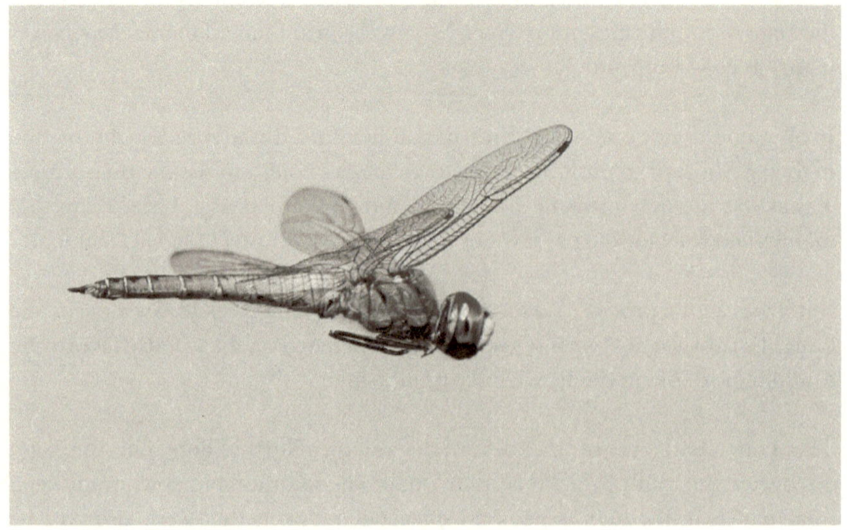

Green Darner dragonfly ~ Dan Graovac photo

The day after Hurricane Henri drenched New England I drove to Crane's Beach expecting to see swarms of swallows preparing to migrate.

But there were half as many swallows as there had been the day before the hurricane. Apparently they had used the calm winds and mild weather of the high-pressure system that had followed the storm to initiate the next leg of their migration south.

But what really caught my attention were thousands of giant, green darner dragonflies, with almost four-inch wingspans. They were so plentiful because the summer's unusual amount of rain had filled the fresh water ponds where they breed.

I could hear the nervous rustling of their silvery iridescent wings as wave upon wave of them flew through the dunes and patrolled the wrackline. They looked so much like a flotilla of tiny hovering helicopters, I found myself quietly humming the theme of *Apocalypse Now*.

I could see their bulbous eyes and clawed legs tucked menacingly beneath their carnivorous mouths. If only there were some greenheads still around so the dragonflies could rip them to bits with their extendable jaws.

But the dragonflies had something else on their minds. After gorging on mosquitoes, midges and sand fleas they would fly down to the tip of Crane's beach and cross over the Essex River to Wingersheek Beach.

They would continue this hopscotch pattern down the East Coast, waiting for propitious weather to help them fly over as much as 30 miles over open water to cross places like the Chesapeake and Delaware Bays.

Eventually they would arrive in Florida and seek out more ponds where they would lay their eggs. Their "children" would hang out in Florida. Their "grandchildren" would hatch out and migrate north and their "great grandchildren' would hatch out of northern ponds and return back 400 miles south again.

It would have taken the dragonflies four generations to complete the round-trip migration, which rivals the better known migrations of monarch butterflies. But their cousins, the wandering glider dragonflies of India, fly even further.

They catch the 3,000-foot high altitude winds that follow the monsoon season then stroke and glide on the winds from India to Sri Lanka and the Maldives. Some of them even use the high altitude winds to migrate 4,000 miles to East Africa, which is twice as long as the migrations of monarch butterflies and several hundred miles longer than Lindbergh's flight from New York to Paris.

All of this is accomplished by an insect that might momentarily rest on your fingertip, if you are particularly lucky.

Ancestors of these dragonflies probably started making these migrations 350 million years ago when India, Sri Lanka and the Maldives were all bunched up together. As the continents drifted apart, the determined little insects just kept expanding their migrations further and further south.

But what has yet to be learned is exactly which organs they use to detect temperature, air pressure, altitude, wind speed and wind direction and how global warming might disrupt their migrations.

But for today it was more than enough to simply marvel at their prowess as the sun set on another gorgeous day in late summer.

CHAPTER 8
Ida, Katrina and Infrastructure
New Orleans
August 29, 2021

In 2005 the United States looked on in horror as levees collapsed, drowning New Orleans under 20 feet of fetid rat and snake infested water. On the exact same day sixteen years later the country waited to find out the fate of the city from Ida, an even more powerful storm than Katrina.

But the country was so fatigued by forest fires, Covid and Kabul that far fewer people watched as Ida slammed into Grand Isle and inched its way toward New Orleans and Baton Rouge.

In 2005 it looked like New Orleans had dodged a bullet the first day after the storm. It was only when an astute observer happened to taste the water leaking through a levee and discovered it was salty, that it became clear that the city would be inundated for several weeks.

One difference was that Katrina had tracked west of the city so the stronger winds on the right side of her eyewall had pushed a much higher storm surge far up into Lake Pontchetrain north of the city. But as the storm passed, the winds changed direction and pushed the storm surge south collapsing the levees and leaving 80% of New Orleans underwater.

However, the most important difference between the two storms was that after Hurricane Katrina the Army Corps of Engineers awarded part of the largest contract in its history to Salem's Bioengineering Group headed by Dr. Wendi Goldsmith.

After graduating from Yale Dr. Goldsmith had attended the Aarhus University in Copenhagen to learn how to engineer cities along biological principles. After receiving her PhD she returned to the United States only to find that there weren't any jobs doing the kind of engineering she wanted to do. So she started her own company, the Bioengineering Group in Salem, Massachusetts.

The Group then won the contract to help shore up New Orleans' three lines of defense: her coasts, wetlands, and levees. They planted trees and grasses and created new islands and the Corps built a two-mile long barrier to prevent storm surges from pushing up into Lake Pontchetrain.

I contacted Dr. Goldsmith the day after Ida and she was guardedly optimistic.

"I can truly say the city's defenses were planned well and built right. Sadly that's rarely the case with large infrastructure jobs that get the common sense whittled out of them due to political pressures and several of the parts will be informally changed along the way."

Would we heed those wise words as Congress debated President Biden's $3.7 Trillion dollar Infrastructure Bill? We can't afford to re-engineer every city to withstand hurricanes and sea level rise. But if we do it right we could potentially create jobs, green energy and use new kinds of cement to actually sequester carbon in newly built highways and bridges.

But we are not going to totally build our way out of this environmental crisis. We have to continue to slow our population growth, reduce consumption and even work less. Several economists have calculated that cutting the workweek to 50 hours would cut carbon emissions in half.

Right now such reductions are being accomplished by Covid-19. We can only hope that our species can learn to control itself so nature won't continue to do it for us in such a Draconian fashion.

CHAPTER 9
Afghanistan
The Saudi Arabia of Lithium
August 30, 2021

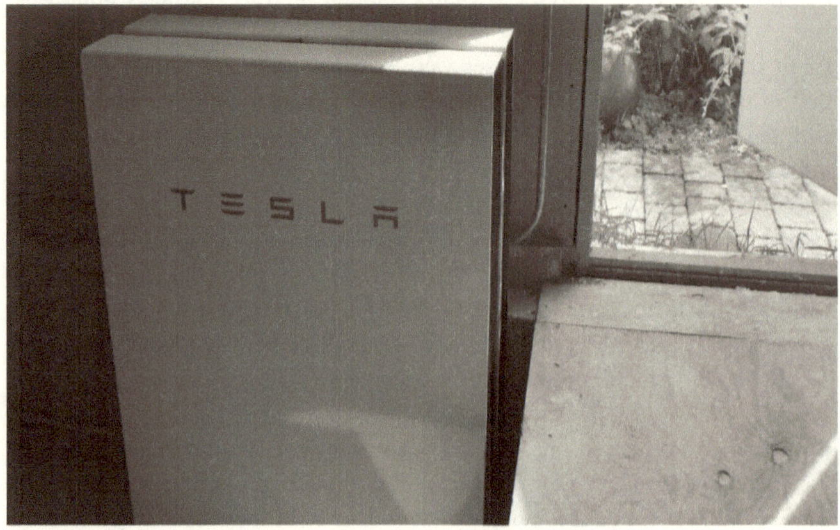

A Tesla Battery

For the past 40 odd years I have been writing about the environmental crisis. But the worst was always yet to come. Glaciers were going to melt, seas were going to rise, storms and forest fires were going to be cataclysmic in 20 to 40 years.

But 2021 was something else. It showed us that we have galloped past multiple tipping points, the apocalypse is now. That realization has put me at odds with almost every news story and economic and political plan I read about. Because if you really think global warming is an existential threat it makes you rethink all your past assumptions.

Afghanistan was a case in point. I disagreed with our decision to invade Afghanistan and Iraq and was happy that we were finally quitting those protracted wars.

But when I realized that Afghanistan has some of the largest sources of copper and lithium I had second thoughts. The world needed those metals if we hoped to avoid the worst effects of global warming.

For example, an electric car requires six times as many mineral resources as a gas fueled vehicle and an offshore wind plant requires nine times more mineral resources than a gas powered plant. And lithium is needed for all their rechargeable batteries and copper is needed to transmit electricity from them.

That is why copper prices were at their highest level in a decade and had they just rose 21% from their price since last July. So this was the result of my new thoughts:

Afghanistan

The United States lost "The Saudi Arabia of Lithium" as Americans prepared for their Labor Day weekend.

Nobody could believe how quickly the Afghan army collapsed. Hadn't we been training them for the past 20 years? Perhaps we hadn't really been training them at all. Perhaps US companies had only been raking in paychecks and construction contracts.

Sure we were there to educate women and keep terrorists in check. But had we also been there to get our hands on Afghanistan's rich supplies of copper and lithium, the two most important ores to fight the effects of global warming?

And now who will get their hands on Afghanistan's estimated $3.7 Trillion dollars worth of valuable minerals? China.

China already uses billions of microchips to churn out digital money that is threatening the world's present financial system and without those chips we can't build and repair computers, cars, I-phones and printers. Now China could forge a monopoly on these crucial metals.

China already has a handhold on Afghanistan's mineral riches through a consortium between the Metallurgical Corporation of China and Jiangxi Copper that has a 30-year on the largest copper mining project in the country.

It spent $3 Billion on the project in 2007 and has included it in its Belt and Roads initiative to help Afghanistan and 70 other countries build roads and infrastructure. In Afghanistan many of these roads will lead to her massive copper and lithium mines.

China already exports more than 85% of the world's rare earth minerals and houses two thirds of the global supply.

We can only hope that China will see that it is in her best interest to keep the price of these metals low enough not to hinder the world's transition to clean energy, or that we have retained enough good will with the Taliban to launch cooperative efforts to mine these metals so crucial to the world's future. But I wouldn't put money on either proposition. It looks like the world is entering a new era dominated by resource wars.

CHAPTER 10
Cruising the Parker River Wildlife Refuge
Newburyport
September 3, 2021

One of the few silver linings of Covid-19 was that it brought about a new reverence for nature. National parks were full, newly minted nomads were trailering across America, folks were flocking to the mountains and sea.

Newburyport is fortunate that it has two areas as wild as the Serengeti only minutes from its urban core. One is the whale and shark filled Atlantic, the other is the Parker River Wildlife Refuge, the main bottleneck of the Atlantic flyway that contains as great a variety of species of migrating birds as any other place on earth. With that in mind I jumped at the chance to join a natural history cruise down the Parker River Wildlife Refuge aboard Newburyport's Yankee Clipper.

Paul Aziz welcomed his passengers aboard and we steamed down the Merrimack against the incoming tide. Fine yachts strained at their moorings and the velvety dark eyes of a seal watched our passage toward the Atlantic. But then we turned suddenly south toward Plum Island Sound.

A large fish jumped near the marsh-lined bank and Captain Aziz explained that it was a sturgeon leaping clear of the water to knock off parasites. The Merrimack used to be so full of sturgeon that some wanted to call it the Sturgeon River, others La Riviere du Gas, fortunately it reverted to its Native American Merriwake, Anglicized to the Merrimack. Good thing too, because the sturgeon were mostly fished out for their roe which was used to replace Caspian caviar.

We continued south with the marshy banks of Plum Island Sound to starboard and the houses of Plum Island to port. It was like the inland waterway that cuts between the barrier beach islands and the marshes of the East Coast from New Jersey to Florida.

We cruised by a flock of cormorants drying their wings and an osprey sitting on a duck blind while her mate chirped and whistled high overhead.

Eventually the houses of Plum Island were replaced by the marsh and drumlin topography of the largest marsh north of New York. Fed by the Merrimack, Parker and Rowley Rivers it has some of the coldest freshest waters of any estuary on the East Coast. This gives her large populations of steamers and stripers but the smallest horseshoe crabs on the East Coast.

Captain Aziz took us through the labyrinth of creeks and pannes, using his twin outboard engines to swivel and turn on a dime. But a few tell-tale bumps on the muddy bottom reminded us that the tide had turned and we must return or be left high and dry in the rich abundance of Great Blue Herons, snowy egrets, swirling swallows and "pee will williting" willets. Not an altogether unattractive proposition.

As we turned, a flotilla of swans ran across the water with the tips of their undulating wings dimpling the surface and their necks outstretched as they slowly lifted and circled overhead, displaying utter disdain for our interruption of their peaceful interlude.

A few more bumps and we ducked under the Plum Island Bridge with its flock of cormorants, commonly called "turd bird" sitting ominously overhead.

Moments later we were battling the outgoing tide and the swollen waters of the rapidly flowing Merrimack River before docking once again. Newburyport, indeed New England, is fortunate to have these two wildlife areas only minutes from its downtown urban docks.

CHAPTER 11
Hurricane Larry; One Strange Bird
Greenland
September 12, 2021

On August 14, 2021, rain fell on Greenland for the first time since the interglacial period 125,000 years ago. Who should worry about that? People in Boston, New York, Miami, Mumbai … even on nearby Plum Island.

The rain was followed a month later by Hurricane Larry that buried Greenland under three feet of snow. Such idiosyncratic storms have become the norm.

Larry started as a West African tropical depression, then quickly become a major hurricane that persisted for 20 days, traveling across the Atlantic to pummel Canada and Greenland before petering out in the Labrador Sea.

Because it stayed mostly offshore, Larry will not go down in the history books. It only knocked out power in Canada and caused two surf deaths in Florida and the Carolinas.

So it was Greenland's rain and melt water that were the real concerns. They highlighted how multiple tipping points can converge to amplify the effects of global warming.

West Coast forest fires had covered Greenland's glacier with so much black soot that instead of reflecting the sun's energy back into the atmosphere, the glacier had absorbed that energy and was melting faster. Plus, the jet stream had bulged south delivering a cold front that had interacted with Larry to create the blizzard.

And it is the melting of Greenland's ice cap that will be the single largest factor affecting sea level rise. This will condemn millions of people to displacement and regular flooding in less than ten years.

Plum Island had a glimpse of that future when Larry teamed up with a high course tide to undermine the island's water mains. Newburyport had to shut off water to three homes to protect the city's idiosyncratic negative pressure waste water system.

Hopefully the measure would be enough to protect the system until the city could install coir bags and the Army Corps of Engineers could shore up the beach with sand dredged from the Merrimack and Piscataqua River in New Hampshire.

The city, state and federal governments had already spent over 25 million dollars to try to slow erosion on the island. The costs would soon exceed the island's tax revenues. Several residents had decided to sell and so far they had always been able to find people willing to buy their distressed properties and build new houses on the same footprint as before. How long can this last? According to glacial geologists, only until 2030... nine years from today, when sea levels will be a foot higher.

CHAPTER 12
A Short Story About a Long Snake
September 15, 2021

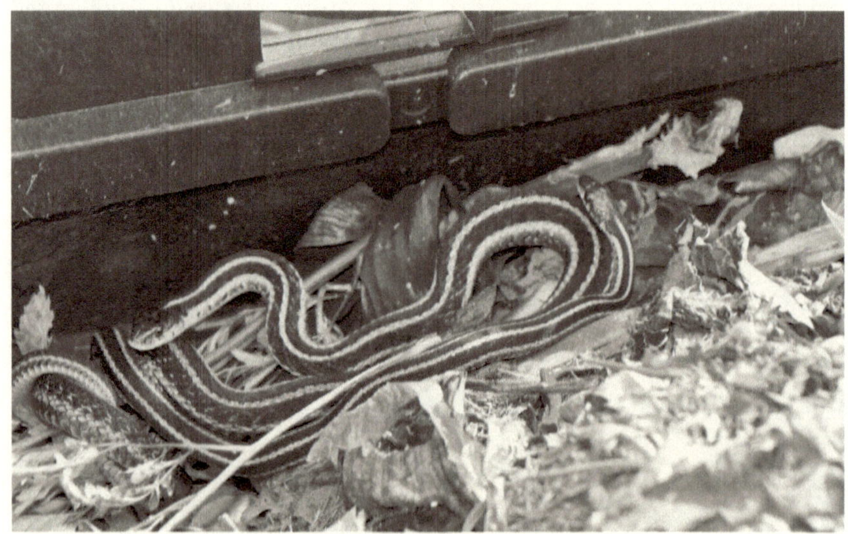

Two mating garter snakes

Every day for the past week I had seen a particularly long and beautiful garter snake resting in my compost bin whenever I lifted its lid.

But my hands were always full so I couldn't get a decent photograph. Besides, I didn't want to disturb his peace and since the only way out of the bin might be to slither up my bare arm I would quietly close the bin and retire.

But on September 15 I decided to solve my dilemma. I quickly removed the cover with my left hand, snapped a picture with my right, and returned my friend to his dark abode.

But when I scrutinized the picture closely I realized I had not seen one long snake with a head on either end but two garter snakes gracefully entwined in startled coitus. Since I didn't want to interrupt said coitus I had quickly shut the lid and departed. Evidently the snakes had been attracted to the warmth generated by the composting litter as the late summer temperatures had started to cool.

When their trysts were over I expected they would be joined by up to a dozen other snakes and use the warmth of my compost bin for their winter hibernaculum.

They are unlike the insectivorous green grass snakes and water loving ribbon snakes that appeared to be more abundant this year because we had so much rain.

As I retreated I thanked them for allowing me a glimpse of their most intimate behavior, wished them good mousing, and told them I looked forward to seeing their progeny in the spring.

CHAPTER 13
Guy Walks Into a Bar... Plankton, Mammoth and Otters
Boston, Massachusetts
September 13, 2021

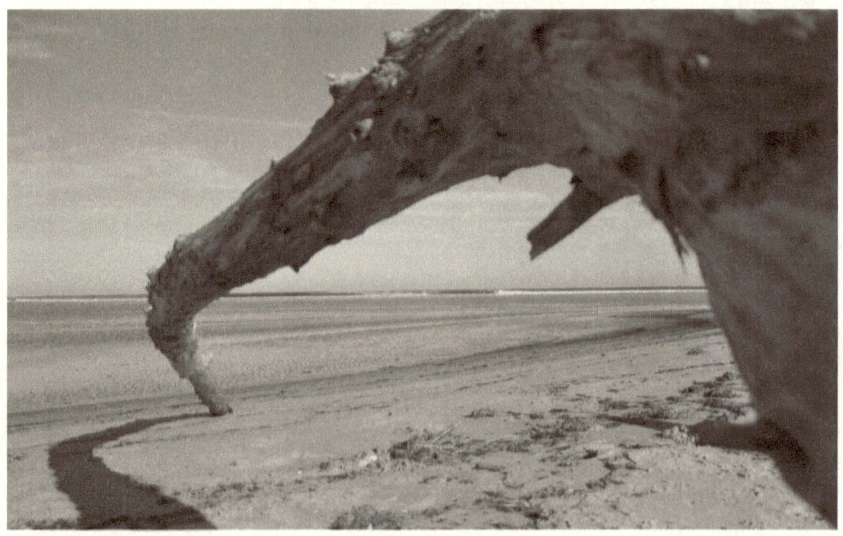

Crane's Beach

On September 13 the New York Times announced that Harvard Medical School scientist George Church had just received $15 million to place thousands of reconstituted woolly mammoth back on the Arctic tundra.

Now if there ever was a problem that didn't need to be solved, this would be it, bring back woolly mammoths to a rapidly warming world? But in a turn of logic as clever as anything the Sackler's used to sell opioids the CRISPR guru justified his scheme by saying that the gene spliced creatures would bring back grasslands by trampling mosses, ripping up trees and leaving mammoth feces all over the melting tundra.

You could say that the brilliant scientist hasn't outgrown what biotechnologists often call their toy stage, the phase where they want to do something really cool with their neat new CRISPR toys. But Church's childlike enthusiasm was so contagious that he was able to raise an initial $100,000 from PayPal's Peter Thiel after Church gave a talk to the National Geographic Society.

But Dr. Church really hit pay dirt when Ben Lamm, the founder of Hypergiant formed a new company called Colossal and capitalized it with $15 million plus seed money from the Winkelvoss twins who lost Facebook to Mark Zuckerberg.

Meanwhile scientists with less access to such luminaries can't get adequate funding to study the humble little planktonic creatures that sequester millions of tons of carbon in the deep waters of the world's oceans every year. Rachel Carson called this carbon pump the most stupendous snowfall on earth.

Anther ongoing project is to bring back sea otters to protect the North Pacific Ocean's kelp beds.

In the 1800's U.S. fur traders were so desperate to find something Chinese merchants wanted to buy that they drove sea otters to the brink of extinction. At their nadir there were only 2,000 sea otters left on the planet.

What happened? The entire ecosystem collapsed. Without sea otters as predators the populations of sea urchins exploded and they, in turn, devastated the kelp beds that are the fastest growing plant species on earth.

Every day kelp grows another two feet and when their fronds die they drift to the ocean floor where their carbon is sequestered for hundreds if not thousands of years.

In 2012 a team of researchers discovered kelp in an area of the Pacific the size of Costa Rica that was capable of sequestering 9 million tons of carbon, which is equivalent to the amount of carbon emitted from a million cars every year.

The same process is also true for eelgrass where sea otters eat the green crabs that feast on the grass. This allows snails to proliferate and scrape epiphytic algae off the eelgrass, so sunlight can illuminate the fronds allowing them to photosynthesize at maximum efficiency.

So far sea otters have only returned to some of their range, there are still 2,500 miles of coastlines that have yet to be recolonized.

Imagine if Dr. Church applied some of his formidable talents to engineering faster growing plankton or found out ways to lithify their calcium carbonate into infrastructure building material plus used some of his $15 million to restore sea otters to the rest of their range. Not as cool as bringing back woolly mammoth but a lot more practical and far easier to accomplish.

Chapter 14
The Crack in Cumbre Vieja
Canary Islands, Spain
September 19, 2021

On 9/11 a swarm of earthquakes started rumbling 18 miles below the surface of the Canary Island of La Palma. Over 25,000 more earthquakes followed before lava spewed out of La Cabezza de Vaca on Sunday September 19.

Serpentine streams of lava were soon snaking their way toward the sea, entombing 300 homes under forty feet of lava and causing 6,000 people to flee. Towering fountains of lava shot 5,000 feet into the air and acrid clouds of sulphur dioxide drifted east threatening the other Canary Islands, Spain, Portugal and the Mediterranean.

The owner of a La Pais jewelry shop recounted "Everything that started on Sunday as something out of the ordinary something beautiful to watch, turned into a tragedy the next day".

But what troubled volcanologists the most was the lengthening rift along the western flank of the Cumbre Vieja mountain range. When I read about the volcano it reminded me that I had first heard of Cumbre Vieja at a seminar about tsunamis like the one that had knocked out the Fukushima nuclear power plant. As the seminar wound down, the moderator asked the panelists, "What would you really like to study if your reputation weren't on the line?"

A well known oceanographer soberly replied, "What really keeps me up at night is a crack in the side of the Canary Islands' Cumbre Vieja mountain chain."

In 2001 two experts on ancient tsunamis, Simon Day and Steven Ward published a paper that warned that a catastrophic collapse of Cumbre Vieja could plunge a 300 cubic mile 1.5 trillion metric ton chunk of the mountain into the Atlantic Ocean. Its impact would then raise a 2000-foot high mega tsunami that would travel across the Atlantic at the speed of a jetliner and crash into the East Coast as a 200-foot high tidal wave capable of encroaching 16 miles inland, inundating cities including Boston, New York and Miami.

The best way to test their hypothesis is to go back into both deep time and deep earth. Two million years ago a super plume of magma rose from the earth's outer mantle to its crust, a distance of 1900 miles. The magma rose as a thin conduit, such conduits can sometimes shoot fully formed kimberlitic diamonds into the air.

As the magma rose it expanded, bubbling out into huge hot blobs that formed mushroom tops as they contacted the mantle, forming 100-mile diameter hotspots. Such hotspots can persist for millions of years. One of the best known of the earth's 17 hotspots formed the chain of Hawaiian Islands; the other formed the geysers and mudpools of Yellowstone Park … and could explode again.

A million years ago the La Palma hotspot broke the surface of the ocean and formed a massive shield volcano. But now all that remains is an empty caldera whose pine tree covered peaks tower a mile over the river filled caldera floor.

The question is, where did all the basalt that used to fit in the mile deep, 5-mile diameter caldera go? It looks like a massive explosion could have blown it into the Atlantic raising a megatsunami, but seismologists believe it washed away over a million years of erosion, making it the largest erosion caldera in the world.

Today the hotspot lies below the Cumbre Vieja mountain chain that runs from the caldera south. This was where lava started spurting out of the rift line of vents on September 19.

Because the lava was hot and fluid it streamed down the mountainside toward the ocean. This is considered to be a "safer" volcano than those that form when one of the earth's plates plunge back into the mantle. Several years ago I visited such a volcano on the beautiful island of Montserrat. The magma was seeping out of the ground with the consistency of toothpaste forming huge unstable needles and caps that caused pyroclastic explosions that sent out shock waves of hot ash similar to the explosions that asphyxiated the people who lived in Pompeii.

So pyroclastic shock waves may not be a problem, but could the volcano break open the Cumbre Vieja rift sliding half the mountain into the Atlantic?

The Cumbre Vieja last erupted in 1949 and 1971. You can still see the two-mile long scars of 40-foot deep lava that flowed down the mountainside entombing houses on its way toward the Atlantic. There are also debris fields where material fell into the ocean and an area in the Bahamas where an ancient Canary Island tsunami might have thrown massive chunks of limestone inland.

But now scientists think that the original paper was wrong and the volcanic material will only slide into the ocean, creating a 130-foot tsunami that would be reduced through bottom friction to a manageable series of 6-foot high waves on America's East Coast. Not high enough to drown cities and wash away homes, however certainly enough to be added as yet another in this year's set of nuisances. At least we can't blame this one on ourselves!

CHAPTER 15
Horseshoe Crabs and Covid-19
Cape Cod
September 20, 2021

On September 20, 2021 John Hutchinson called to tell me he couldn't find any small horseshoe crab shells in Cape Cod's Pleasant Bay. This was disturbing, but not unexpected.

Horseshoes have been harvested from the bay for the past 40 years. Their strikingly beautiful blue copper based blood is worth $1,500 a quart and is used to test for bacterial contamination.

But since the pandemic, demand for the valuable animals had surged. All the vaccines and antibody tests used to fight Covid-19 had to be tested with a preparation of horseshoe crab blood called Limulus amoebbocyte lysate or lysate for short.

Normally the ancient creatures shed their shells every year and the empty shells end up tangled in the wrackline by late summer. For years my friend George Buckley had his Harvard students count the number of horseshoe crab shells along a 100-meter transect in early September.

But in 2000 he told me, "Bill the population of horseshoe crabs has crashed in Pleasant Bay. We can't find any immature molts."

"But George", I said, "the bay is choke full of large female crabs."

He told me my writing stunk and I told him his field technique was no good. But we finally decided to figure out what was really going on.

We measured the width of 500 adult crabs and observed where the fishermen were collecting and returning them. We discovered that up to 250 crabs died from the bleeding and handling process. Good collectors could make over $100,000 a summer, but they had to catch 400 unbled crabs a day. This became more difficult as the season progressed.

By the end of the summer up to 90% of the bay's 100,000 crabs would have already been bled, so the collectors started to collect the female crabs when they came inshore to lay their eggs.

However, the Cape Cod National Seashore owns these waters and it is illegal to make a profit from animals captured in a national park. The Seashore was embarrassed when they realized the collectors had been catching crabs in their waters for the past twenty years. They banned the practice, George and I published our results and the Seashore won a federal court case in 2000 to uphold the ban.

We argued that collecting the large females had removed them from the breeding population so that the number of immature crabs had declined. But we didn't realize just how right we were.

The following summer we counted 200 to 300 molts along the 100-meter transects. The year before George's students had only counted 2 or 3 crabs. The ban had worked far better than advertised.

I kept on seeing 200 to 300 crabs until Covid hit and demand soared. The collectors were hard pressed to harvest 400 crabs every day so they had apparently reverted to their old ways, sneaking back into the shallow waters while the crabs were mating under the new and full moon high tides.

What could the Seashore do, chase them with pursuit canoes?

The collectors had several incentives for skirting the law. The country was in the midst of a medical emergency and the bleeding companies were stretched thin trying to meet demand. But they had an additional incentive. A researcher in Singapore had used gene splicing to develop an artificial form of lysate that did not require using live horseshoe crabs.

The FDA didn't want to switch horses during the pandemic. They had 30 years experience using the cheaper more sensitive natural lysate but only two years of trials with the new synthetic version, so they turned it down.

But the writing was on the wall. Everyone expected the synthetic lysate would be approved after the pandemic quieted down and the multi-million dollar lysate industry would come to a rapid end, along with its lucrative horseshoe crab fishery.

Perhaps the companies could justify sacrificing a year's worth of horseshoe crabs because once the synthetic lysate was adopted the 450 million year old species would have another million years or so to recover. I wonder about our own species.

CHAPTER 16
"Regular Gas, $3.42"
The Energy Crisis; Hamilton, Massachusetts
October 13, 2021

Just when the world appeared to be emerging from Covid-19, an energy crisis emerged at the worst possible time.

The Glasgow Climate Conference was just three weeks away. It was supposed be the time when the world would finally turn irreversibly away from fossil fuels and toward a future of clean, green, renewable energy.

But the world seemed to be recovering from Covid faster than expected and winter was not far behind. Demand for oil, gas and electricity had soared and governments responded by turning back the clock.

China's President xi-Jinping had said he intended to close down China's coal plants, but reversed himself and ordered them to increase production to a whopping 100 million metric tons. President Biden had petitioned OPEC to increase the production of oil to drive down the price of gas in the U.S. and Europe was turning away from its Green New Climate Deal.

Climate change had ironically been part of the problem. There had been less rain in China so her hydroelectric plants had produced less electricity so she had turned back to coal. There had been less wind in Europe so her wind turbines had produced less electricity so she had turned back to oil. Plus Russia had slowed gas exports to European countries to force them to approve Gazprom's Baltic Sea pipeline to Germany.

China was not alone. The United Kingdom had reactivated an old coal plant and other countries were keeping coal and oil plants open way past their expiration dates.

Just to top things off, a container ship had ruptured an old oil pipeline off Huntington Beach, California. It was eerily reminiscent of the 1969 Santa Barbara spill that was the most dramatic and highly visible catalyst that had spurred President Nixon and Congress to pass more environmental bills than any other time in our nation's history. They included such signature pieces of legislation as the Clean Water Act, the Environment Protection Act and The Endangered Species act.

It also helped spur Wisconsin's Senator Gaylord Nelson and California's Senator McCloskey to organize Earth Day, which attracted more than 20 million people.

So perhaps the past two years of forest fires, heat waves, storms and now an oil spill would spur Congress to pass president Biden's climate agenda and make the Glasgow Conference a success. But is massively rebuilding the infrastructure of China, Europe, Russia and the United States the best way to reduce humanity's impact on our finite world?

CHAPTER 17
Sequestering Carbon, Nature's Way
The Matthew's Estate; Hamilton, Massachusetts
October 18, 2021

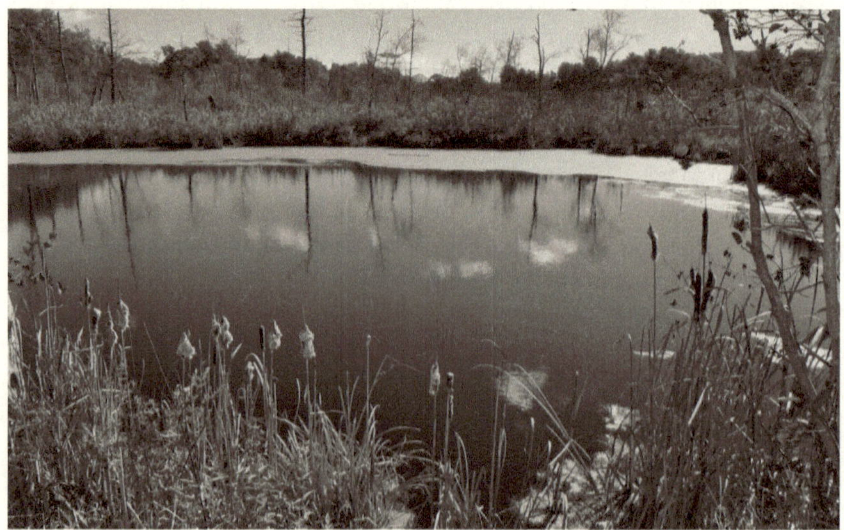

Mathews Plantation

Trees are nature's way of sequestering carbon and the best place to see how this works is the Harvard Forest in Western Massachusetts. But when I started to research the early history of the forest I was surprised to learn that it included one of the earliest and most extensive experiments in conifer cultivation and it was right next door in Hamilton Massachusetts. It is the 99-acre Mathews plantation given to Harvard University in 1929 by Nathan Matthews, then the Democratic mayor of Boston.

The university established the forest to serve its forestry students, in the same manner as teaching hospitals serve medical students, by introducing the latest European silviculture practices "to supplement the old pioneer psychology of prodigal waste".

The Forest's Fisher Museum in Petersham shows the history of that typical New England forest that returned after the glaciers scrapped off previous forests. That set the scene for the succession of soft and hardwood forests that would follow.

The museum's opening diorama depicts the 1700 pre-settlement Petersham forest. The Nipmuc people were already using forest products and burning underbrush to make it easier to hunt deer, turkeys and bear. At this time the landscape was 90% forested with only a few clearings for growing corn, squash and beans.

The second diorama shows the same landscape in 1740 after European settlers forced the Nipmuc off the land and cleared the land for larger fields and pastures.

The peak of deforestation occurred from 1830 to 1880. During that time the situation had reversed and only 10% of the land was forested and 90% had been cleared for agricultural purposes. All that remained of the forests were 10-acre woodlots the farmers used to heat their homes.

All the bear, deer, turkeys, beaver and wolves had disappeared or retreated north. It was during this pastoral period that Thoreau marveled that someone had seen a deer several towns over. Other than that, the largest wild mammals he ever saw were muskrats and grassland birds like meadowlarks and bobolinks were common.

During the Civil War, New England farmers were exposed to the deep rich mid-Western soils. They had responded by returning home and abandoning their rock-strewn fields for the more tillable soils of the mid-West. Fast growing white pines reclaimed the New England fields and their canopies blocked sunlight from reaching the hardwood saplings living in their shadows.

By 1900 Yankee entrepreneurs started clear-cutting the white pines, which opened up the canopy to fast growing hardwoods like red oak, red maple, white ash and birches. Their canopies blocked the sunlight so white pines couldn't get reestablished in turn. The first person to recognize and name this process as succession was Henry David Thoreau, whom I like to think of as the reigning science writer of his time.

Armed with this knowledge I tried to find the Matthews Estate. It was not an easy task. The Estate did not advertise itself. The only sign was a 2-inch trail marker tacked to a tree that said Harvard Forest and the remains of a granite pillar and stone wall that had once marked the entrance to the coach road that led into the estate which they called a plantation at the time.

But once I was on the trail I could see the old stands of pine trees and hemlocks that used to be the most dominant conifer species in New England. In recent years hemlocks have been decimated by woolly adelgids. US Forest Service scientists predict that the sap-sucking insects will affect Southern forest carbon cycles, but these plantation trees seemed remarkably healthy and lacked the fluffy white egg clusters of the adelgids.

The Cutler Pond showed the greatest change. Chinese rhododendron had gone wild but they still delineated the banks of the old pond but beavers re-introduced into the reforested area had converted the pond and surrounding lowlands into an extensive fresh water marsh.

All that remained of the conifer farm was a ghost forest of hundred foot tall white pines that had died when the dammed up water had drowned their roots.

The only open part of the pond was covered in duckweed. But you could see that it was filling in and as time passed the pond and marsh would turn into a dry pasture and be reforested again. So today areas like the Matthews Forest are more natural than at any time since the American Revolution.

During the last three hundred years the succession of such New England forests have sequestered over a quarter of a million tons of carbon and if we preserve them they will continue sequestering millions more. That would be the equivalent of taking 15,000 carbon spewing cars off the road.

By the same token, if we harvest the forests sustainably and use their trees for lumber they will continue to keep carbon out of the atmosphere, and prevent emissions from high carbon producing building materials like steel and concrete. Compare this natural process, which is almost free, to the industrial removal of carbon that costs $600 a ton.

63

Chapter 18
Sequestering Carbon, The Industrial Way
Iceland
October 25, 2021

Several years ago I was invited to tour a dozen Swiss firms that were involved with Green Technology. They were doing things like improving wind and solar energy, and investigating ways to make low carbon cement.

But the most far-fetched idea was being noodled around in Zurich's Climeworks company. They were proposing building thousands of machines to suck carbon dioxide out of the air. At the time it was just a gleam in their geo-engineering eyes.

But now their second plant named ORCA has come online, near Iceland's Central Rift Valley. This is where a warm spot has lifted the mid-Atlantic ridge above the ocean floor. It is also where basalt is seeping out of the earth pushing the Atlantic plate west and the European plate east.

It is this fresh basalt that is an integral part of the intriguing project. Powered by Iceland's abundant geothermal energy, giant fans suck carbon dioxide out of the atmosphere, filter it, heat it with water and pump it down into the reactive basalt, which cools the slurry and converts it to limestone over the course of two years.

The limestone will sequester the carbon dioxide within the earth. Theoretically it could also be used to make limestone blocks to build limestone houses similar to those on Bermuda.

So far the process is being done on a minuscule scale. The ORCA plant pulls 4,000 tons of carbon out of the atmosphere, which is the equivalent of the carbon emitted by 790 automobiles, compared to the 575 tons of carbon sequestered by a hundred acre forest like the Mathews conifer estate in Hamilton. But the big difference is that using this industrial method, it costs $600 a ton to remove the carbon while nature does it for free.

ORCA's costs will come down but Climeworks estimates they will have to build half a million such facilities to remove our annual rate of carbon emissions.

Somehow it reminds me of the New Year's Day film *The Time Machine* based on the novel by H. G. Wells. In the film, pollution has destroyed the earth and humanity has evolved into two species. The pastoral Elois live an idyllic but vacant life on the earth's surface, that looks a lot like Southern California, and the Morloks who slave underground running giant fans to suck air into their underground lairs. They only came out at night to snatch and eat the unsuspecting Elois.

Not a very appealing vision of the future. Iceland's carbon sucking machines may solve part of the sequestration equation but nothing beats the natural carbon sinks of our oceans, forests, trees, marshes and peatlands. And nothing beats keeping carbon spewing fossil fuels underground in the first place.

Chapter 19
Methane; Glasgow's Key to Success?
October 22, 2021

As the diplomatic world inched closer to the Glasgow climate summit the natural world took another hit. Gazprom, the Russian oil and gas company, admitted that it had caused the biggest methane leak in two years.

It happened in June when a broken pumping station leaked 2.7 million cubic meters of methane, the global warming gas that is 86 times more harmful than an equal amount of carbon dioxide. Scientific American has described methane's action as warming the planet on steroids.

The announcement could not have happened at a worse time. Gazprom had been counting on natural gas being the transition fuel for the developed world as it weaned itself away from coal and oil. Instead the industrial world was retreating from green energy just as Gazprom was trying to force Europe to approve its pipeline to Germany.

But then the European Space Agency's satellites had detected huge plumes of invisible methane spewing out of the Yamal pipeline in Siberia.

The Energy consultant company Kayrros estimated that the pipeline was spewing out 93 British tons of methane every hour which was equal to the amount of yearly carbon emissions from 15,00 cars.

Formerly, carbon estimates had been based on calculation of the amount of carbon dioxide pouring out of tailpipes and smokestacks.

But as satellite technology improved researchers discovered that leaking oil and gas pipelines and pumping stations were emitting far more methane than originally thought.

This was good news for cows. It meant that their farts only accounted for 25% of the world's methane emissions and mud volcanoes and natural gas seepages accounted for even less. Nature was off the hook.

Companies like BP and Royal Dutch Shell invested in their own satellite companies so they could repair their leaks and stick by their pledges to cut methane gas emissions.

The results of the satellite surveillance were impressive. In 2019 satellites discovered a pipeline leak in Turkmenistan that was repaired, removing emissions produced by the equivalent of a million cars.

But the really good news about methane is that it could be the key to rapidly and inexpensively reducing the rate of global warming to under 2 degrees Celsius.

On September 17 the U.S. and Europe pledged to reduce methane emissions 30% by 2030. It followed Trump's veto of a former pledge by the U.S., Canada and Mexico.

The reason that policy makers were so encouraged by the action was that methane only stays in the atmosphere for a dozen years, so such cuts would be quickly apparent, as opposed to the effects of carbon dioxide cuts which can take many decades to notice.

If the U.S. and Europe can convince other major methane emitting countries like China, Russia and India to join them, the world could start seeing rapid positive results in the health and well being of themselves, their children and their planet.

CHAPTER 20
Think Global, Act Local
Washington D.C.
October 29, 2021

President Biden glanced at his watch. In only a few hours he had to fly to Rome then on to Glasgow. He still didn't have the votes he needed to pass the Bipartisan Bill that would give him something to say at the conference. All because of that damn senator Joe Manchin trying to save his dead coal industry in West Virginia.

This meeting had been Biden's last-ditch effort to convince house democrats to pass the bill that would pledge $500 Billion to help America switch to electric cars and utilities to convert to renewable fuels.

It was not as if other countries had much to offer either. Covid and climate change had thrown spanners into the mix. China was reactivating its coal plants, Russia was pressuring Europe to accept its gas line to Europe. India was refusing to pledge its carbon reductions because it said it hadn't caused the problem.

Diplomats were mouthing the words that Glasgow was our last best hope, but everybody wanted to do it on the cheap. They were being fed the myth that you could just rebuild the infrastructure, switch fuels, buy a fancy new electric car and continue with their all-consuming energy wasteful ways.

My generation had come of age reading *Silent Spring*, *The Population Bomb* and *Limits to Growth*, books that presented what I still feel is a more clear-sighted view of the environmental crisis and what we need to do to reverse it. Stop producing synthetic chemicals, stop having so many children, use far less total energy and stop runaway economic growth on our fragile finite world.

Many of my contemporaries made substantial lifestyle changes. We didn't follow our parents into corporate America but moved to rural places like Alaska, Oregon and Cape Cod to live more simple, environmentally friendly lives. We mixed our new environmental ethic with the traditional hunting and fishing conservation ethic. We helped improve the lives of many small towns and villages in these areas and provided impetus for the many pieces of Sixties and Seventies legislation that form the underpinnings of today's environmental laws.

The Glasgow Conference reminded me of the 1974 Law of the Sea Conference I attended in Caracas as a representative for the Sierra Club. The attendees included some of the most learned scientists, lawyers, diplomats, marine experts and industrialists in the world. Many had spent the bulk of their careers working on developing a treaty to structure the governance of three quarters of the world's surface.

After several years of preparatory meetings and wrangling, this conference finally came up with a well-crafted treaty. What happened? During his first week in office President Reagan vetoed the bill. Diplomats saw the last twenty years of their careers go up in smoke.

It was then that I decided to return to my roots — to think globally but act locally. To concentrate on saving the bay I had grown up on, protecting the animals I loved and working with local groups, to solve solvable local problems rather than insolvable international ones.

And what did countries do after the Law of the Sea Conference failed? They returned to their roots and set about establishing national territorial limits, exclusive fisheries zones and forging regional agreements to manage their mutual marine resources.

It was a reminder that the history of UN climate and population conferences has always been a history of failure. That is why the 2015 Paris Agreement included a ratcheting mechanism so countries could increase the size of their carbon cutbacks every 5 years.

After the Paris Agreement the executive director of the world coal association told the Financial Times that the agreement had not heralded any great changes. But he was wrong.

Technological advances in the energy sector had caused coal consumption to drop 10% below where experts had expected it to be. Similar changes were happening with oil and gas.

If countries ratcheted up their emissions pledges at Glasgow, it would undoubtedly accelerate the process. But if they didn't, it wouldn't be the end of the world. It wouldn't be enough to reverse the economic momentum to switch to cheaper renewables.

So far nations were holding their hands close to their chests. We would have to see what the next fortnight of negotiations would bring and whether it would be enough to convince nations to ratchet up their carbon cutbacks before we rush past several more tipping points in our onward rush toward environmental catastrophe after environmental catastrophe.

Chapter 21
Sharks and Seals; Worms and Coronaviruses
Cape Cod
November 3, 2021

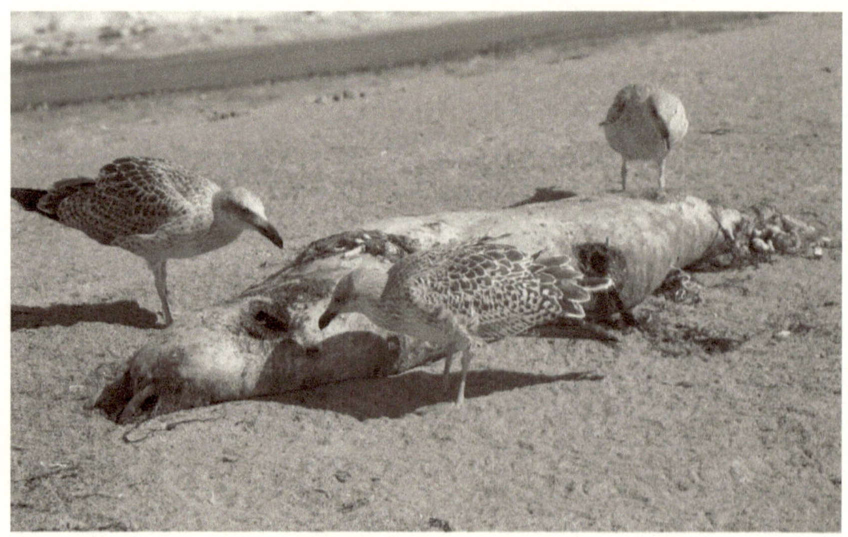

Seals killed by Morbillivirus

In 1995 wildlife managers reintroduced wolves into Yellowstone National Park. It had been 70 years since the apex predators had been extirpated from the area.

But by 1998 the wolves had culled the moose and elk populations, eliminating over browsing by the voracious herbivores. This caused a resurgence of other species including buffalo that had been out-competed for food by the hungrier elk.

Soon beavers returned along with frogs, snakes and wetlands invertebrates. Finally scavenger species like grizzly bears, bald eagles and ravens that depend on wolf kills returned to their former abundance along with six species of songbirds that bred in the restored wetlands vegetation and the willows, aspen and cottonwoods that all the other species depended on.

We are conducting a similar experiment on Cape Cod but it comes with several interesting twists. The first is that Atlantic cod that live near Grey Seals are extremely "wormy". They can contain encysted and wriggling nematodes whose eggs had been excreted by the nearby seals, then eaten by euphausid shrimp and passed on to codfish, which if eaten can cause life-threatening anaphylaxis in humans.

It is also pretty disconcerting to see worms rearing their heads like miniature cobras, so don't expect to find cod sushi at your local sushi bar. Just the sight of a wormy fillet of cod is enough to make most buyers shy away from such infected fish.

During the Sixties, states like Massachusetts and provinces like Nova Scotia paid fishermen bounties to kill seals. They thought the seals were eating too many codfish and they felt that by getting rid of seals they could get rid of the nematode worms as well.

Then in 1972 Congress passed the Marine Mammal Act, and what happened? Seals rebounded and along with them came a resurgence of their apex predators, Great White Shark who are so myopic they often mistake human swimmers for seals.

Grey Seals have responded by changing their behavior. So instead of migrating through sharky water they have taken up year-round residence on places like Nantucket's Muskegat Island whose surrounding waters are so shallow the sharks can't ambush the seals from deep water.

The other twist is that seals harbor coronaviruses similar to those that cause Covid-19. They are in the Morbillivirus family and can infect dogs, cats, cattle, whales and humans. The most common Morbillivirus is canine distemper followed closely by phocine or seal distemper.

The most recent phocine distemper outbreak occurred in 2018. Plum Island and Crane's Beach were strewn with dead and dying seals and over 3,000 seals died up and down the North Atlantic coast.

The alarming thing is that the virus can be transmitted both vertically from mother to infant and horizontally from one species to another so seals could act like an amplifier organism for potential human outbreaks. This puts Great White sharks in a different light. They are crucial to the health and productivity of the oceans including their seal and codfish populations. We are but fleeting visitors in sharks' realm. It is we, not them, that have to be careful when we swim in their natural feeding territories.

CHAPTER 22
Shark Attack!
Sandy Point
August 15. 2018

When I took photos of a decomposed seal on August 15, 2018, I assumed it was one of the seals killed by a virus. But after I posted the photos Mike Morris sent a photo of the same seal taken from three days before my photo.

You could see several large shark bite marks on the body and see where the shark had crushed the seal's ribs. Then the shark had torn off the seal's head leaving only the lower jaw behind. Mike said the bite marks were similar to ones he had seen from attacks in the area before. It just goes to show you usually see what expect to see, not what is really there!

Several years before a fisherman was standing in the water watching a seal play off Plum Island's North Point when a shark attacked the seal sending the fisherman clambering up the steep dune in his bulky waders, all to the delight of the other fishermen on the beach, who didn't believe him. They made him the butt of their jokes until several more seals were found with similar bite marks from a Great White Shark.

Mike was something of a shark attack expert himself. Early one morning he was surfing off Plum Island when a Great White Shark had bashed the bottom of his board leaving teeth prints that matched the size of those found on dead seals the following day.

And a few days before I had taken the photo of the dead seal two paddle boarders had been cavorting with some Humpback whales as they fed on menhaden in front of the houses on Plum Island. Right in the middle of this feeding frenzy was a large triangular dorsal fin. Local experts insisted it was the fin of a basking shark, but that didn't make much sense. Basking sharks feed primarily on plankton. But guess what? Menhaden are one of Great White Sharks' favorite food items.

The same day I took the photos a man was standing in the water 30 yards off Cape Cod's Newcomb's Hollow Beach when a shark tore into his torso. He was rushed to the hospital where he presented in good condition, but was later downgraded to fair condition. That afternoon fishermen reported seeing a Great White Shark in the mouth of the Merrimack River.

All these sharks had probably been born in a Great White Shark nursery ground off New York City, which somehow seems fitting. About 20 years ago one of the young female sharks from the nursery swam north and discovered nice fat gray seals rolling around in the shallow waters off Chatham. She started preying on the seals and news of the new food source spread by word of mouth, as it were. The seals were plentiful because the Marine Mammal Act had made seal bounties illegal. Formerly fishermen had been encouraged to kill the seals because they were a vector for cod worms that went on to infest the flesh of codfish making it unmarketable.

But global warming has heated the ocean temperatures enough so that menhaden now swim regularly north around the biological barrier we call Cape Cod. We had seen the results all summer. The water temperature was about seven degrees higher than usual and Right, Humpback and Minke whales were feeding just off the beach beside striped bass and tuna that were also feeding on the now abundant menhaden. The larger fish had trapped the menhaden against the shore and chased some into fresh water rivers where the menhaden had died from lack of oxygen.

The Great White Sharks are perched at the very apex of this food pyramid. They were feeding on the seals, striped bass and menhaden and were not above taking an exploratory nip out of an occasional human swimmer. This is what happens when you throw nature out of whack. She fights back to reestablish a new equilibrium under the different, new conditions.

CHAPTER 23
Sequestering Carbon; One Whale at a Time?
Salisbury, Massachusetts
August 22, 2019

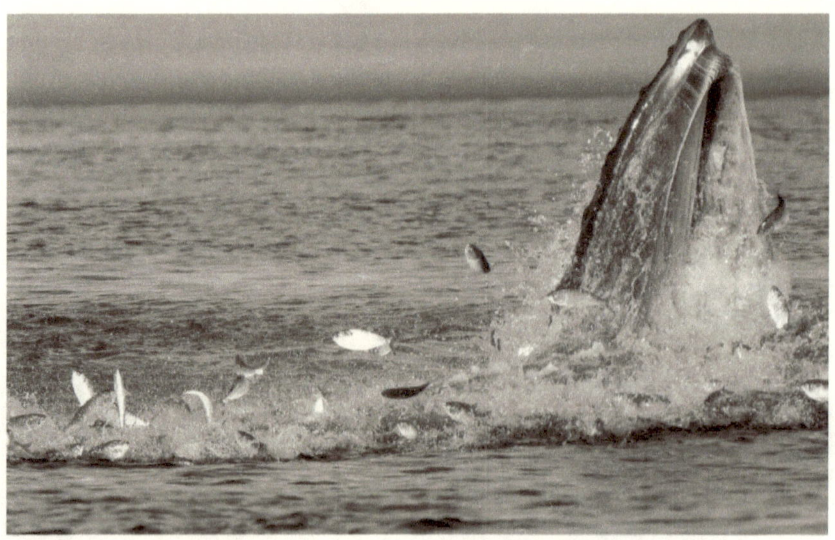

Capturing carbon one whale at a time ~ Dan Graovac photo

Excitement rippled up and down the Salisbury Beach in 2019. Storms had piled up water along the shore and humpback whales were lunging through thick schools of menhaden. They surfaced with their huge mouths full of the silvery fish that leapt into the air and spilled back into the water.

Each fish weighed over a pound, so the whales were swallowing hundreds of pounds of fish every time they lunged and they would lunge up to 500 times a day. So by the end of the day, they would have swallowed up to ten tons of food. That's the equivalent of 70,000 Big Macs, or equal to the amount of calories I have eaten during my entire life. It makes me a little ill just to think about it!

The whales' food chain is one of the shortest and most efficient in the animal kingdom, from plankton, to menhaden to whale blubber in just a few short days.

But, here is where it gets really interesting. What happens after a whale eats the equivalent of 70 thousand Big Macs? Whale size poops! And it turns out those poops are chock full of iron which is considered to be a rare commodity and a limiting factor to phytoplankton productivity in the open ocean. But the whale's fecal plumes spread iron nutrients close to the sunlit surface waters where they get snapped up by phytoplankton which are fed on by menhaden and krill and are eaten again by whales.

Before large baleen whales were decimated over the past two centuries, they annually recycled 12,000 metric tons of iron every year. Today they only recycle 1200 metric tons.

Researchers think that historically whales maintained plankton feeders like menhaden and krill. But today populations of krill have drastically declined and some researchers would like to fertilize the ocean with iron to increase phytoplankton and in turn increase species like krill to ultimately increase the numbers of baleen whales.

The other thing you do when you add iron to the oceans is sequester carbon as the phytoplankton sinks to the ocean floor.

On the face of it this form of geo-engineering might seem like a good idea. But adding too much iron to the oceans holds the potential of creating blooms of Pseudo-nitzshcia, phytoplankton that can cause amnesiac shellfish poisoning. This is what made San Francisco's sea lions so aggressive and arguably insane several years ago.

Chapter 24

Building Our Way out of the Environmental Crisis; Will it work?
Washington D.C.
November 5, 2021

"Beware: Gaia may destroy humans before we destroy the world."

~ James Lovelock, 2021

Congress finally passed President Biden's $1.2 Trillion dollar Infrastructure Bill on November 5. Six Progressive Democrats voted against the bill because it didn't include the Build Back Better economic package that would have provided $555 Billion dollars to move toward renewable energy. To their credit, thirteen Republicans voted for the bill thus overruling the Progressives brinkmanship.

Most of the dissenters from both parties came from contentious places like Massachusetts, New York and New Jersey.

The bill had something for everyone. High speed railway systems spidering out from San Francisco and Los Angeles to California's economically strapped Central Valley, $7.5 Billion to build charging stations so California drivers, who own 40% of the Teslas in the country, could recharge their batteries while driving from San Francisco to Los Angeles.

Cities like Boston and New York would finally be able to eliminate their Amtrak maintenance backlogs and the state of Wyoming would be able to fortify its avalanche prone highway over the Teton Pass. Oregon would be more secure that a major earthquake wouldn't collapse their Vancouver to Portland Bridge and Californians would be aided by well paid federal wildfire fighters, while Alaska would get $250 million to develop electric ferries to transport passengers to its isolated and far-flung wilderness communities.

Sixty-four billion dollars would be used to upgrade the nation's broadband system and refurbish transmission lines, so Texas would not be crippled again by the recent blizzard that froze her many wind turbines.

What was missing from the bill was the $555 Billion dollars in the Build Back Better act that would cut back 1000 metric tons of carbon emissions by 2030, the equivalent of taking a year's worth of cars and trucks off of American highways. It wouldn't be passed before the end of the Glasgow Conference but Congress hoped to pass it by November 15.

In essence The Infrastructure Bill was really just a massive jobs program. Like many environmentalists I remain skeptical that we can build our way out of the environmental cull de sac we find ourselves in without making real sacrifices, but it had the excitement of FDR's New Deal. At least we were doing something.

The pandemic had just shown us that, echoing the words of James Lovelock, if we don't do something, nature will destroy humans, before humans destroy the world.

CHAPTER 25
The Healing
November 18, 2021

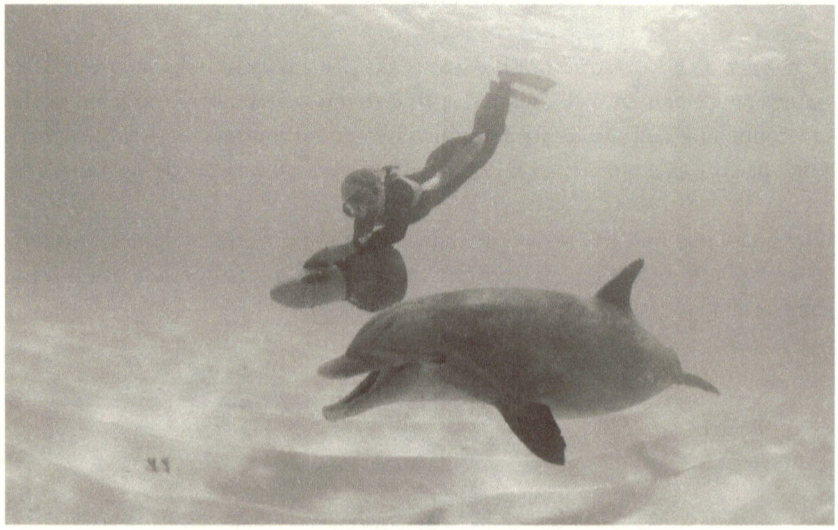

Jay swims with the Patriarch ~ Ethan Daniels photo

On November 18 the Discovery Channel drove me to Rhode Island to film a segment with my sister Jay. I could get used to this!

Jay is one of those remarkable women who have a unique bond with wild animals. I have seen a young moose come out of the woods and start nuzzling her parka as she spoke to him in an adoring yet authoritative voice. When we filmed her walking into her barn twenty horses came to attention as she told them how handsome they were.

For twenty-five years my sister has also been part of a pod of wild dolphins and special friends with its patriarch, who is himself unique among his species.

Somehow in the vastness of the ocean this remarkable woman and this remarkable cetacean have found each other and forged an unbreakable bond in the Bahamian Islands.

Today this bond is particularly poignant because my sister has inoperable cancer and the patriarch is himself old and covered with scars.

Jay has to have regular chemo sessions and undergo dialysis three times a week. However she still wants to visit her patriarch friend so he can introduce her to his latest offspring. He has taught one calf how to approach humans, perhaps in preparation for becoming the next ambassador to our terrestrial species.

Just as the patriarch has introduced my sister to his family, my sister has introduced her husband, daughter; sister and me to the patriarch and I don't doubt that the patriarch knows exactly how each one of us is related to his special friend.

In addition to being such empathetic social beings, dolphins also have the ability to use their sonar to diagnose and heal disease. Mother dolphins scan their nursing infants with pulses of sonar to see if they are having gastronomical problems. If she detects a bolus of gas she will caress the spot to release the gaseous pressure.

The first time I met the patriarch my back was in pain. Just floating weightless in the warm alien world made me feel better and I found I could exercise strenuously without irritating my back. This was fortunate because the pod was swimming particularly fast that day.

But the patriarch suddenly turned and floated vertically in front of me. He stared fixedly into my pain filled eyes, then abruptly scanned me with a burst of sonic pulses. It felt like a physical therapist had just passed an ultrasound wand over the precise disc that was bothering me.

We know that dogs can use their keen sense of smell to sniff out skin cancer in humans and nip off any lesioned cells. I like to think that after my sister and the patriarch reunite and tell each other about their lives and families that the patriarch will bath my sister in a soothing shower of sonar pulses to draw out the illness lurking in her plasma cells.

It is such interspecific bonds and strong friendships that give me hope that we can somehow heal our polluted planet. If we don't, I fear future Cetacea will warn their great grandchildren to avoid any species with our long, grasping, acquisitive fingers and curiously large hypertrophied brains.

CHAPTER 26
Resource Wars; Cobalt
November 23, 2021

For more than a century the world has been enmeshed in an ongoing petroleum war. The United States, Great Britain, France and the Netherlands created companies like Aramco, British Petroleum and Royal Dutch Shell and backed them up with diplomatic and military power to carve up the Middle East into vassal state oil reserves. This led to a hundred years of bitterness, colonialism, greed, wars and terrorism.

Now, with lightening fast rapidity, we find ourselves in the midst of an equally deadly battle ignited by the world's perceived need to build batteries, microchips and electric cars. The two prime combatants in this new resource war are China and the United States. In early 2021 we saw China's Belt and Road Initiative serpentining toward Afghanistan's recently vacated lithium mines.

The next battlefield will be the cobalt mines of the Congo, where China has already stolen a march on the United States. While both the Obama and the Trump administrations stood by, China's government backed company, China Molybdenum, bought two Congolese cobalt mines from the American firm Freeport McMoRan that simply packed up and left the Congo for good. Freeport had once been the largest cobalt producer in the Congo, the country that produces two thirds of the world's supply of cobalt. Now the International Energy Agency expects a cobalt shortage in 2030, other experts suggest it will be as soon as 2025.

Now the Biden Administration is trying to negotiate for supplies of cobalt from Australia and Canada, but it is clearly a case of closing the barn door after the horse has fled.

But it had always been a surprise hiding in plain sight. After President Obama and Xie Jinping agreed to cut carbon emissions prior to the 2015 Paris Climate Conference, China prepared a comprehensive playbook detailing how it planned to dominate the world's clean energy economy.

While the hard-hatted Donald Trump was stomping through West Virginia promising coal miners "You are going to be working your assess off once I'm elected". China Molybdenum was purchasing the Congo's Tenge Fungurume mine that produces more cobalt than any other country on the planet. Trump further advanced China's ambitions by rolling back U.S. requirements to accelerate the transition to electric vehicles.

A few years later China Molybdenum purchased the Kinsange mine which has the capacity to produce batteries for hundreds of millions of Teslas.

The transactions caught the Biden administration off guard, as it had been when it realized that China had plans to take over Afghanistan's lithium mines in the wake of the United States precipitous withdrawal.

It was suddenly clear that China had beaten the U.S. in the latest round of the New Great Game to monopolize the world's resources for the transition to green energy. To add to the urgency, in August 2021 China Molybdenum announced it would increase production to 40,000 tons of cobalt. In 2020 the U.S. had only produced 600 tons. China had already announced it would provide Congo with $6 Billion dollars to build roads hospitals and schools in exchange for ten million tons of copper and 600,000 tons of cobalt.

But Congolese villagers know that when the new blasting starts, the walls of their mud framed homes will crack, chemicals will seep into the rivers where the women do their laundry while watching out for hippo attacks and eventually the mine will announce that everyone will have to relocate, similar to when the United States mined Congolese uranium to bomb Hiroshima and Nagasaki. Would these be the similar downsides of the world's efforts to build its way out of its environmental crisis?

CHAPTER 27
The Glasgow Fiasco
Scotland, UK
November 14, 2021

The United States climate envoy John Kerry entered the plenary hall with his right arm draped over the shoulder of his Chinese counterpart Xie Zhenhua. Their masked faces hid the fact that Europe, China and the United States had just dashed the hopes of First World nations, developing countries, island nations … the world.

Billions of people had been shafted as the world's four largest carbon emitters had caved in to India's demand that the final text be changed from saying that the countries had agreed to "phase out" coal, to they had agreed to "phase down" the use of coal.

The other signatories were incensed. It was going to be the first time that any international climate agreement had even mentioned coal, the fossil fuel most responsible for global warming and the big four had watered the text down to near meaninglessness.

In the year that had seen deadly heat in Canada, drowning floods in Germany, killing fires in California and horrific hurricanes in America's Southeast, the conference had only come up with a modest agreement to reduce methane, meager funds from rich countries to poor countries to transition to renewable energy and minor progress on setting up carbon markets, all way short of the overall goal of keeping the rate of global warming below 1.5 degrees Celsius.

As disappointed as delegates were, the last year of environmental calamities and Glasgow's minimal achievements had been a wake up call. The world now knew how difficult it was really going to be to get wildly different countries to act together to solve an almost intractable global problem.

At the Paris Conference in 2015, nations had agreed that they would return with new pledges for reducing emissions in five years. Nothing said that the Glasgow Conference had failed so miserably as delegates' realization that now they would have to return with new pledges every year if they hoped to reduce their carbon emissions. It was not a pretty sight, but the world finally had a more clear-eyed view of the problem—if not its solution.

CHAPTER 28
Oysters; Ocean Acidification Threatens One of our Proudest Industries.
Ipswich, Massachusetts
December 14, 2021

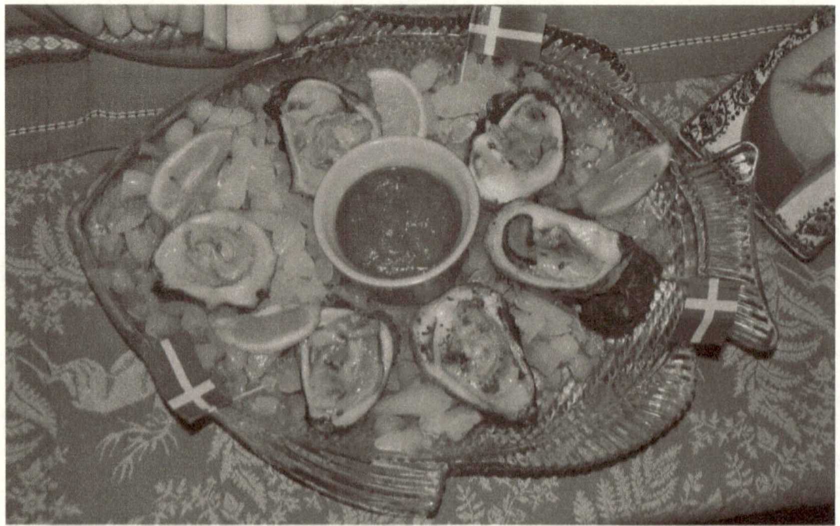

Ocean acidification threatens our oyster dinners

Shellfish have a long history of helping people pull themselves up by their bootstraps. In 1819 Thomas Downing, the son of a former slave moved from the tidewaters of Virginia to New York City where he established the Downing Oyster House. It soon became famous for serving such celebrities as Charles Dickens and sending oysters to Queen Victoria.

Downing realized he could transform New York's popular black run oyster cellars from places of ill repute, usually across the hall from bordellos, into well-adorned restaurants where a gentleman could feel comfortable bringing his wife. Still a little louche but with far better décor.

It was to pursue a similar story that I drove to Eagle Hill to scratch up my Christmas oysters. Trucks and trailers were converging on the landing and clambers jostled and bantered as they backed their trucks into the water to launch their aluminum skiffs.

Their forefathers had used sailboats and rowboats to gather the oysters that would be loaded onto railroad cars and shipped throughout the land. "Eagle Hillers" were considered to be some of the best oysters in the country because of their succulent flavor, from fresh water and mud, la gout du terroir of the Ipswich flats. If you struck gold in San Francisco the first thing you did was to order a bushel of "Eagle Hillers" and a magnum of brut champagne.

During the depths of the depression George Pappas founded the Ipswich Shellfish Company. His ancestors had been recruited in Greece to work in the Ipswich textile industry and been issued signs that were pinned to their jackets saying Ipswich Mills. After the recruits were processed at Ellis Island the signs helped get them directed to the right trains and transportation to Ipswich.

In Ipswich they lived in company houses, bought food in company stores and were paid far less than their English-speaking counterparts. When the non-English speaking workers struck for higher wages, police were brought in and deliberately fired into the picket lines, hospitalizing many strikers and killing a young girl who was simply watching the proceedings from the sidewalk. The Mill owners tried to pin the blame on the prominent Pingree family who had helped organize the strike.

The Spanish flu and the depression had added to the community's miseries. But George Pappas saw a way out. In 1935 he founded the Ipswich Shellfish Company that paid fishermen a good price for their shellfish and delivered their produce up and down the East Coast. No longer tied to flat wages, the fishermen could make good money for honest hard work — almost as much had been made doing slightly less honest prohibition work.

Today the Ipswich Shellfish Company owns six companies from Maine to South Carolina and employs hundreds of people that dig, shuck and sell shellfish across the country. Money made from scratching up the valuable bivalves has also supported two beautiful churches, the elegant and festive Hellenic Center and numerous well-situated homes, an all-American up by your bootstraps kind of story.

Oysters; Ocean Acidification Threatens One of our Proudest Industries.

But today that industry is threatened by ocean acidification. When you try to shuck an oyster its calcium carbonate shell often crumbles in your hands. Yet another industry that has given pride to a whole community is now threatened by what we have done to our atmosphere and oceans.

CHAPTER 29
"Like a Big Bomb"
Mayfield, Kentucky
December 11, 2021

America was enjoying the shoulder season on December 11, 2021. Despite vaccinations, the number of Covid cases was about what it had been at the same time the year before. Deaths were over 800,000. But the fires, heat waves, floods and storms of summer had passed. The South and Midwest were enjoying unseasonably warm weather. It was 79 degrees in Memphis, which broke the record set a hundred years before.

Warm moist air spawned in the Pacific by La Niña and steamy hot air flowing off the overheated waters of the Gulf of Mexico had nestled into plains and valleys. Drier cooler air was blowing rapidly overhead. The conditions acted like a chimney, creating a path for the heat and humidity to spiral furiously upwards in a series of fifty odd tornadoes.

Some congregated into a massive tornadic thunderstorm that carved a 250-mile path of destruction from Arkansas through Missouri, Illinois, Tennessee, Ohio and Kentucky. It sucked the whirling remains of farms, homes and factories 30,000 feet into the air and lasted for more than three hours.

Inside the Mayfield candle factory, workers were working 24/7 to meet holiday demand. Elijah Johnson asked his foreman if he could go home after the tornado siren sounded at 9 pm.

"You can't leave. You can't leave. You have to stay here. If you leave you will lose your job."

"Even with weather like this you're still going to fire me?"

"Yes!"

Some workers left anyway so managers took a roll call to figure whom to eventually fire.

Those who remained took shelter as the lights began to flicker. Pressure built up until people's ears popped as if they were on a crashing plane. Then the building collapsed like a pack of cards. Kyanna Parsons-Perez found herself pinned under 5 feet of debris and enveloped in darkness. People were starting to panic, so she told her colleagues:

"Tomorrow gonna be my birthday. Y'all gotta sing Happy Birthday to me."

Strained voices started singing the familiar words but others cried out in fear.

"I couldn't move anything. I couldn't push anything I was stuck." Kyanna told NBC news.

Rescuers had to crawl over corpses to reach those still trapped but alive in the rubble.

With deaths approaching ninety bodies spread across five states the tornadic thunderstorm would go down in the record books as the deadliest December tornado on record, probably the most deadly in any month. The previous December tornado had happened in 1953 when 38 people were killed in Vicksburg Mississippi.

The big question on everyone's mind was, is this the new normal? It's complicated. While it is fair to say that atmospheric conditions created by global warming can support cool season tornadoes, as yet there is not enough evidence to show that the number of strong tornadoes is any different today than it was a hundred ago.

More evidence would come when the weather struck again three days later. On December 15, torrential rains and blizzards blasted across the country and into the mountains from the West Coast to the East. Tornadoes and Derecho straight wind storms flipped tractor-trailers on their sides and skidded them across the highway, at least one dead driver was trapped inside.

Hurricane force winds touched down in 55 places setting the record for most hurricane force gusts in a single day.

However, the most frightening statistic to emerge from the 2021 data, was that the temperature had soared to over a hundred degree Fahrenheit in Verkhoyansk Siberia. Hundred-degree weather is easier to grasp than the goal of limiting global warming to 1.5 degree Celsius. It is something even the most ardent climate change denier has trouble explaining away.

CHAPTER 30
Fusion; Energy's New Hope?
MIT
December 1, 2021

"None of us is trying to win trophies, we're just trying to keep the planet livable."

~Maria Zuber, Vice President for Research, MIT, 2021

December 1 was a clear cold day. People couldn't believe the world was about to enter the third year of the Covid epidemic. They couldn't believe the Glasgow conference had been such a disaster. They couldn't believe we would have to endure yet another year of environmental catastrophes. We seemed to have entered yet another long gray winter depression that wouldn't go away.

But the Wall Street Journal dropped a bombshell of optimism into this cloudy cauldron of gloom. It announced that an MIT spinoff company called Commonwealth Fusion Systems had raised $1.8 billion to develop nuclear fusion technology. Two of the financial heavy hitters were George Soros and Bill Gates.

However, the real watershed moment had come four months earlier as the result of an undergraduate project that proposed using long flat tapes of barium oxide superconducting material to build a super magnet capable of creating a magnetic bottle of wispy ions heated to over a hundred million degrees Fahrenheit, the equivalent of creating a small star.

On September 5, 2021 they had ramped up the magnet as a series of steps until it reached the goal of a 20 Tesla magnetic field. Many experts think this could be the critical step that would lead to a limitless supply of safe, clean nuclear energy.

The next step will be to build SPARC, their prototype power plant that will shoot deuterium and tritium atoms toward each other at over a million miles per hour. This would be enough to fuse them together releasing helium and gigawatts of clean energy. The only fuel would be water, and safety should not be a concern because as soon as power is shutoff the plasma instantly dissipates, without releasing any radiation.

What made this revolutionary new advance possible? The long thin tapes containing rare earth barium copper oxides that make the magnets powerful enough to make small safe fusion power plants that are able to yield more energy than they consume. And Commonwealth Fusion Systems plans to complete SPARC in only four years.

Like MRNA technology that made all the new Covid vaccines possible, Commonwealth Fusion Systems says competing entrepreneurs will also be able to benefit from their rare earth barium oxide technology.

As if to blunt the impact of the Commonwealth financial announcement, the day before, British Columbia's General Fusion announced it had raised $130 million from Jeff Bezos' venture capital fund Bezos Expeditions. It would help them build their own demonstration fusion plant outside London. Earlier China had announced it had heated up its Tokomak artificial fusion apparatus to 270 million degrees Fahrenheit, ten times hotter than the sun.

Despite the gamesmanship of competing press releases it is clear that the race to produce fusion energy was heating up. It would all be based on rare earth barium copper oxides and where do they come from? China that had the foresight to monopolize the minerals that would fuel the new green energy market. It was already processing the majority of the barium, lithium, nickel and cadmium being used to transition to a new world order powered by safe, clean green energy. Will China dominate renewable energy the way Western powers have dominated the old world order based on oil?

CHAPTER 31
The Pipeline
January 12, 2022

They come in long gray rows, the caravans of oversized trucks that pull into the Green Plains ethanol plant in Central Nebraska. Workers open chutes in the bottoms of the trucks and streams of golden corn kernels cascade into an underground chamber where a conveyor swept them up to the top of a growing mountain of golden corn. Only this corn is not destined to feed pigs, cows or chickens, it is destined to feed our desires to drive gas-guzzling cars.

The problem is that producing ethanol also produces carbon dioxide, but now 31 of those Midwestern plants plan to pressurize that carbon and pump it through a network of pipelines to North Dakota where it will be sequestered permanently underground.

It would be like taking 2.6 million cars off the road and will keep ethanol competitive in California, Oregon and Washington that have passed regulations that require purchasing gas with lower carbon footprints. The 315-mile pipeline will cost $4.5 billion and create thousands of construction and dozens of permanent jobs.

Of course pipelines have a bad reputation thanks in part to the Keystone Pipeline project. But pipelines are not the problem it is what's in them that is. In this case there won't be any tar sands or oil to spill and ignite.

In fact pipelines are about the safest way to transport most gases and liquids. I was reminded of this several years ago when landowners were protesting against a proposal to build a pipeline to pipe natural gas to a New England power plant that wanted to switch to gas that was twice as carbon free as oil and would supply electricity to 1.5 million homes. Most of the protesters feared the pipeline would lower their land values.

The protest got me thinking. As a kid I grew up in Dover, Massachusetts. You might have heard of it. Boston Globe columnist Mike Barnicle used to chide

Dover for its mile-long driveways and having more trees than people. It was not known for its low land values.

When I was about seven, Algonquin Power laid a natural gas pipeline behind our house. I imagine everyone was compensated for the use of their land. I just remember walking my dog through the woods to watch the huge excavators connect and bury the sections of pipes. I must admit I was also intrigued with the idea of the pipeline snaking its way all the way back to the Gulf of Mexico.

But after a few weeks, the excavators disappeared and everything went back to normal. The scar over the pipeline gradually healed to become a nice broad path that wove its way through the thick woods. The only problem that I was able to unearth about the pipeline was that someone had found some invasive plants growing along the woodsy pathway.

Other than that, the pipeline was so well forgotten that neither Dover's town clerk nor its conservation agent were aware that the pipeline even existed. Presumably all this time the pipeline had been transporting millions of cubic feet of gas without incident. So much so, that by 2014 Massachusetts was producing 60% of its electricity from natural gas plants.

So, perhaps the only good thing about last year's weekly drum roll of heat waves, forest fires, freezes and floods is that they were impossible to deny, and that people, countries and companies are starting to figure out what they can do to lower their carbon footprint.

Some of the proposed solutions are high tech, others are low. Some will have unintended consequences others will not. Some are quite literally outlandish ideas; others make good, down to earth, common sense.

Removing carbon dioxide from ethanol and sequestering it underground is one of those good middle tech solutions that could make a lot of sense, if we decide to continue using ethanol in our gasoline.

CHAPTER 32
Manganese Nodules; Cobalt for the Future?
The Clarion-Clipperton Fracture Zone
January 22, 2022

One of my first jobs was working at the Caracas Law of the Sea Conference for the Sierra Club with funding from a Quaker group. It was my way of avoiding Hanoi University but that is a story for another time.

The problem with the job was that while the Sierra Club wanted to protect the oceans, the Quaker group wanted me to lobby delegates to create something called the Enterprise, an international entity established to exploit deep-sea mining "for the benefit all mankind".

I was reminded of that compromising job when I investigated how the successor to the Enterprise, the UN's International Seabed Authority is now promoting seabed mineral mining.

Housed in a nondescript building in downtown Kingston, Jamaica, The International Seabed Authority is supposed to both protect the deep ocean but also manage seabed mineral mining. It is the classical example of the fox guarding the chicken coop.

The authority worked just fine as long as nobody had the money or interest to mine the ocean floor. Some of the world's leading scientists and lawyers had been bamboozled because everyone thought Howard Hughes was about to make billions of dollars mining manganese nodules. It turned out later it had all been a cover-up for a CIA operation to raise a Soviet submarine. That too is a story for another time.

But now multinational companies realize that someone really can make billions of dollars mining cobalt from the seafloor, rather than having kids dig it by hand in places like Congo and Afghanistan.

The area that is most likely to be developed first is the Clarion-Clipperton Fracture Zone that stretches halfway across the Pacific from Hawaii to Mexico. Its abyssal plains are littered with billions of nodules. They look like deep-sea potatoes but are million year old conglomerates of magnesium, iron, nickel and cobalt.

Promoters say the nodules can be the answer to how we are going to manufacture all the cobalt-based electronics, batteries and electric cars that will usher in the new era of sustainable green energy.

But the best way to see the Clarion Clipperton fracture zone is through the eyes of Diva Amon, a Trinidadian marine biologist.

Diva won The International Seabed Authority's award For Excellence in Deep Sea Research in 2018 but now the British Museum of Natural History scientist is caught in a dilemma.

When she descends in a submersible to explore the Clarion Clipperton Fracture Zone she sees anemones with eight-foot long tentacles, sea cucumbers that look like cuddly teddy bears, sharks that glow in the dark and glass sponges that have been around since the Stone Age. Ninety percent of them are entirely new to science.

That's the problem for Dr. Amon and the handful of scientists who have actually explored the area, "We don't have enough science to make informed decisions about how to manage this activity." Because of comments like those, the ISA no longer invites Diva to their workshops on environmental management of the deep seas.

For years marine scientists have been calling for a moratorium on deep-sea mineral mining to give researchers time to clarify the potential harm of such mining and how to mitigate its impact. The head of the ISA, British lawyer Michael Lodge calls their proposal for such a moratorium, "anti-science, anti-intellectual, anti-benthic development and anti-international law".

But scientists counter that scrapping the ocean floor could permanently affect their communities. But they fear the greatest impact could be from plumes of sediment caused by dumping mining tailings back into the sea. The toxic tailings could kill off zooplankton over large swaths of the Pacific Ocean and clog up the biological pump that sequesters millions of tons of carbon every year.

Proponents argue that land based mining for cobalt could lead to a greater loss of species. But ultimately it comes down to whether you think we should engineer our planet for the benefit of one species, ourselves, or for the benefit of the interconnected web of organisms that make up our life supporting biosphere.

It is clear that the biosphere can exist quite happily without our species. The question is, can we exist without the biosphere? About the only person who thinks we can is the uber Star Trek fan Elon Musk.

CHAPTER 33
The Island
12/21/21

Stegner (not his real name) looked out at the pathetic looking seawall in front of his house. It was a Rube Goldberg combination of two 15-foot long sand bags made of biodegradable coconut fiber held in place by thick wooden poles sunk 10 feet into the sand. Plus a wall of boulders trucked in from a quarry somewhere up in Maine.

The wall was already collapsing and they hadn't been any storms. The high tides had simply washed through the boulders and pooled up in front of his house. Each wave then sucked more sand from behind the seawall further eroding the beach.

The jury-rigged seawall had already created another hotspot of erosion, as had every other anti-erosion device built on the island in the past sixty years.

First it had been groins that cut off the flow of sand, then sand bags that had washed away, seawalls that had collapsed, then the rebuilt jetty that stopped Stegner's end of the island from growing. Each scheme had been hailed as a success; each had failed and increased erosion. Each had been the result of political maneuvering to figure out what could be done. Nobody had paused to consider what should be done.

Stegner knew what should be done; return the beach to what it had been when he bought the house. Then, his neighborhood had been nestled amongst thirty-foot high sand dunes so far from the shore you couldn't see the ocean and the beach had been growing robustly then.

Now what you would have to do was lower the jetty, remove the jetty spur, open up the groins and tear down the seawalls so the island could move, pulsate and grow again like it did when he was a boy.

Sea Level Rise might wash away a few more houses, but more would be lost by erecting more seawalls and building houses on the same footprint as before.

All it would take would be half a dozen guys armed with crowbars on a moonless night. Rumor had it that people had done similar things on the other end of the island but Stegner was too decent to break the law.

He had built this house to enjoy his retirement, now it all it was doing was ruining his health and making him miserable.

What did it matter if a glacier was poised to collapse somewhere in the Antarctic Ocean anyway? Removing the anti-erosion devices would keep his island healthy if he was lucky. After that what would he care? Stegner would be dead.

CHAPTER 34
The Emergency!
January 28, 2022

"What we need is for the Governor to declare an emergency, right now!"
~Tom Saab, Salisbury resident, 2022

There was fear and anger in the Merrimack River Beach Users Alliance zoom meeting on January 28. It had been scheduled as a regular meeting of residents and local officials but it had become an emergency meeting to deal with a bombogenesis storm packing hurricane force winds, 18-foot waves and a 9-foot high tide.

Stan Sacks' home had been condemned and 18 others damaged by a much less powerful storm two weeks before. It was clear that the Rube Goldberg seawall that had been cobbled together after local officials found a loophole in the state's regulations wasn't going to protect homeowners any more during this storm than the last.

Newburyport police chief urged everyone to evacuate. Formerly officials had told residents to use magic markers to print their social security numbers on their wrists so they could be identified after they drowned. Apparently they had been told to cool their rhetoric this time. The head of the DPW announced that several electric and sewer lines had already been cut off because they would be so covered with sand after the storm that workers couldn't find the lines. If the sewer lines broke the whole system could go down, leaving basements and bathrooms filled with putrefying sewage as had happened in 2015.

The Fire Chief announced that a fire truck and an ambulance would be stationed on the island, and Ron Barrett of the Plum Island Tax Payers Association announced that their PITA Hall would have food and heat for anyone caught by the storm.

"But we can't take pets because we don't want dogfights or anyone getting bitten along with everything else!"

Senator Tarr closed the meeting by exhorting everyone to stay safe and work together to survive what was expected to be an historic storm.

The Storm: January 29, 2022

New Englanders can be pretty damn smug about global warming. After all, we don't have out-of-control forest fires, killer heat waves, deadly tornadoes and destructive hurricanes. But Massachusetts has more major storms than any other East Coast state, how come?

The answer was raging right outside my window, a bombogenesis Northeaster ready to coincide with a 9-foot high tide, 18-foot waves and hurricane force winds. In the summers we get hurricanes, to give us more storms that any other East Coast state.

The big question for this storm was whether the 2-foot storm would coincide with the 8 o'clock high tide.

The storm had been dubbed Kenan. Don't you hate these winter storm names? It started at midnight with high winds and snow but by 6 AM there had been little accumulation and no hurricane force winds.

A Boston news station is airing a story about a Cape Cod house in danger of tumbling off a cliff in Truro. Nantucket is expected to go underwater during high tide and the owner of the Graves Lighthouse in Boston Harbor is hunkering down with his fishing buddies to enjoy their homemade Portuguese stew.

What New Englanders do get is this front row view of sea level rise, the fastest horse in the environmental apocalypse. Every year, every storm, hell, every high tide changes a beach and the barrier beach I had watching most carefully for the past ten years was Plum Island. There, people had built groins, seawalls and jetties, just about everything you could possibly do wrong to a barrier beach, and each had created a hot spot of erosion just downstream of itself.

THE EMERGENCY!

Two weeks before, the much less powerful storm had led to 18 damaged homes. Another had to be condemned after local officials had found a loophole in the state's regulations that allowed them to throw up the Rube Goldberg design that combined the worst features of both a seawall and a fortified sand dune.

Most of the residents believed that the seawall had saved their homes. But the problem with seawalls is that waves accelerate as they crash through the wall of boulders, which causes the waves to scour out a slurry of sand behind the seawall so it collapses landwards. This is what happened to the house that had to be condemned, its foundation had cracked as it slumped into the water filled sand.

The problems had all arisen when residents in the center of the island had convinced the Army Corps of Engineers to rebuild a jetty on the Merrimack River in the mistaken belief that it would slow erosion almost a mile away.

What it had done was block the natural flow of sand to the beach in front of the houses at the north end of the island. They had lost 400 feet of high dunes and beach in six years. The same thing had happened the last time the Army Corps of Engineers had rebuilt the jetty. But what had happened? The Blizzard of 1978. It had broken up the jetty so sand could flow through again and the beach had grown 400 feet back again in under six years.

Residents had been hectoring the Army Corps of Engineers to lower a section of the jetty to create a weir, but it would probably take ten years to get through the Corp's tangle of red tape. But the Blizzard of 1978 had solved the problem in under 36 hours. I couldn't wait for the storm to pass so I could get out there to see if this storm had caused the jetty to settle and solve the residents' problems yet once again.

CHAPTER 35
Aftermath
Plum Island
February 2, 2022

The twin memes that stuck in everyone's heads after the January 28 storm were the students paddling down Nantucket's flooded streets in blowing snow and the house in Truro hovering miraculously on six spindly four by fours above the raging Atlantic.

The owners were trying to get permission to move the house onto an empty lot owned by the Cape Cod National Seashore. They didn't have very much time. A third storm was due to arrive on February 3.

The first thing I wanted to see was how the south jetty of the Merrimack River had fared. As I struggled over a snow covered path I could see that water had covered most of the beach and that the jetty had settled another inch or so.

But the jetty had not been totally disheveled as it had been during the Blizzard of '78. Another 6,000 cubic yards of sand had flowed through the jetty, but as long as the spur of the jetty remained the sand could not accumulate in front of the houses on Northern Reservation Terrace. Unfortunately, nature had not saved the day. Humans would have to try something else.

I trudged back to see the houses close to low tide. I could see that waves had over-topped the seawall and pushed a lot more sand and water against the houses, but miraculously less damage had occurred in this storm than during the less powerful storm two weeks before. Evidently the strongest wind had blown on either side of high tide.

Soon people were flooding social media demanding that more boulders be added to the Rube Goldberg seawall. But it was clear that things had gone too far. There was not enough beach and the energy was too strong. No amount of rocks was going to be able to save the situation. In fact if more rocks were added to the seawall they would just accelerate waves causing them to undermine the houses more quickly than before.

Nobody wanted to admit it, but homeowners' best bet would probably be to follow the example of the Truro family and move their houses back from edge. It would be expensive but you would still have your house on the ocean for as long as it would take for the Army Corps to fix the jetty. One family had quietly done that on Plum Island and they could safely expect their home would remain just across the street from the ocean for the next generation of owners.

There were several empty lots behind the houses on Northern Reservation Terrace, several of them on the same street as their present location. Moving the houses to those lots would allow the owners to continue to live in their own houses on the island until the Army Corps of Engineers could fix the problem, if they chose the right solution.

CHAPTER 36
Could Seals Harbor the Next Pandemic?
Ipswich, Massachusetts
02/02/22

On February 2 my cozy little 2-room apartment filled up with lights, cameras, diffusion screens and a camera crew. Irene Von Schyndel and I had spent the day before cleaning and scrubbing to make my humble little workhouse presentable.

I love its light and simplicity. It makes me feel like I'm on a boat. The sun rises on one side of my room and sinks on the other. Space is so tight you have to keep everything shipshape and orderly which is damn difficult for writers.

Decorations are few: horseshoe crab molts, driftwood, a frieze of blue mussels lined up a ledge with the sun shining through deep green wine bottles.

Fortunately my rescue plants were all in bloom for the shoot. Pink and red geraniums reached for the sun on the tips of long thin teleolated stems. Boston park workers were going to throw the plants out at the end of the summer and seemed happy I could offer them a good home.

The geraniums were offset by multiple blossoming poinsettia plants. I had bought them for two bucks ten years before. One was 5 feet tall but it had started to develop aphids so I had to put it outside where its shriveled up branches silhouetted in the snow made me feel like I put down the family dog. I had found the avocado plants sprouting in my compost heap and now they were over four feet tall as well.

After a few hours of setting up equipment we were ready to roll. The producer, David Roolhoof, asked me about a recent book I wrote about the origins of Covid-19. It had been the first book to investigate whether the pandemic had been caused by a lab accident. But I also gave credence to the idea that the disease could have spilled over from nature.

I was curious why David had started with this question. It didn't really seem relevant to a film about sharks and seals. I was more comfortable when we started talking about how "wormy" codfish and seals are, and how states like Massachusetts had used bounties to keep the numbers of seals in check so more codfish would be available to fishermen.

But because seals were vectors for codfish worms the bounties had the added benefit of reducing the number of the unsightly parasites. I described collecting the worms from newly gutted fish much to the consternation of the wealthy boat owners.

But we went on to discuss when corona-like viruses had decimated harbor seals in 2008 and 2018. I had seen where coyotes had come down to the beach at night to feed on the rotting carcasses. This had exposed the coyotes to the seal distemper, which is close to coyotes' own virus for canine distemper.

We discussed how dogs, cats and pets like hamsters have contracted Covid-19 along with all the gorillas in the San Diego zoo. Plus the millions of mink that Denmark euthanized because they had contracted Covid.

It was clear that most of these animals had been infected by human contact, even when the humans had been wearing personal protective equipment.

Spillover usually happens between closely related species but that is not always the case. Flu viruses can infect such species as humans, pigs, sparrows and whales. This gets us back to seals.

Up to a third of the Grey Seal pups on Nantucket's Muskegat Island are infected with corona-like viruses. Most of the pups probably picked the virus up from their mothers but where did the mothers get the viruses?

Some scientists think that California's Elephant Seals picked up H1N1 influenza from wastewater during the 2009 swine flu epidemic.

It turns out that testing wastewater is the most effective way to determine the number of Covid cases before patients have started exhibiting symptoms and before health care professionals have even reported the cases.

COULD SEALS HARBOR THE NEXT PANDEMIC?

Water is supposed to kill viruses but when you have billions upon billions of virions in a wastewater stream who is to say that a few wont be viable enough to infect a seal swimming through that water or breathing the virion filled air just above the surface? As everyone's favorite skeptical scientist says in Jurassic Park, "Life always finds a way".

But what about Covid-19 spilling over in the other direction from wild animals to humans? This could be humanity's greatest risk.

Viruses need two types of hosts to thrive and multiply, reservoir species and amplifier organisms. Part of the reason many scientists were skeptical that Covid had spilled over from bats is they couldn't identify an amplifier organism in which the viruses could mutate and become more contagious.

Now we have millions of superabundant amplifier organisms including deer, seals and ourselves. There are a number of things we can do to handle the seal situation. One would be to amend the Marine Mammal Act, which was intended to protect whales, but because seals are marine mammals they were included as well. The human situation will be a lot more difficult to handle.

But before we handle that conundrum, let's look more closely at another amplifier organism, the elegant but way overpopulated white-tailed deer, and their parasitic sidekick, the black-legged tick.

CHAPTER 37
"Do you have a problem with that … Deer?"
Covid-19 and Climate Change
Ipswich, MA
February 10, 2022

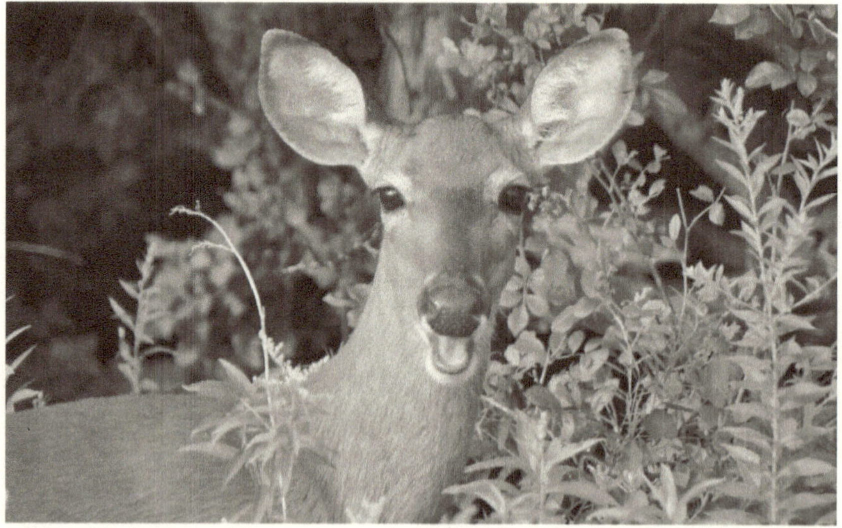

This deer is covered with ticks and was coughing for several days

There are 30 million white-tailed deer in the United States. So far the U.S. Department of Agriculture has found Covid antibodies in deer in every state it has tested in. Their results range from 19% of the deer testing positive in New York, 31% in Pennsylvania and 67% in Michigan.

It is yet another example of the unexpected consequences of tampering with nature. In the case of seals it was the Marine Mammal Act that led to the overabundance of seals and now to the overabundance of their apex predator, the Great White Shark.

We also know that deer populations have exploded since we wiped out their apex predators wolves. We used to think that their range increased when farmland turned back to forests after the Civil War. Now, however, scientists believe the reason that deer have moved north and become so abundant is because of climate change. Warmer winters have allowed deer to expand into boreal forests and find food while avoiding snowy cold winters where they can be worn down and killed by coyotes, which are not as big and as good hunters as wolves, but are starting to take over as deer's' apex predators.

Frankly, it is difficult to explain why so many deer have contracted Covid-19. They have little contact with humans other than being shot. There are a few farms that raise deer for venison but they are few and far between. I know of people who feed deer but most of them have stopped for fear of spreading Lyme disease.

However Chinese scientists have unearthed DNA evidence that suggests that Omicron originated in mice. And deer are infested with ticks that transfer diseases between mice, deer and humans. So deer could have contracted Covid from ticks that had been on mice that go live in people's houses during the winter then transfer Covid to deer through their tick vectors when they move out into the surrounding fields in the summer. Not a very appealing thought.

Once a deer contracts Covid it is easy to see how they pass it on. They are herd animals and the herds intermingle in and out of the rutting season.

Unfortunately this gives us a glimpse of our planet's possible future. We have systematically created superabundant species like seals, deer, sharks, ticks and ourselves.

In doing so we have created the ideal conditions for a whole host of infectious agents. They exist like bombs timed to mutate and explode into repetitive cycles of globe girdling pandemics on a planet consumed by heat, humidity, illness and pestilence; unfit for mankind but congenial for species still not yet evolved to destroy their own biosphere.

CHAPTER 38
The End of Barrier Beaches
Plum Island
February 16, 2022

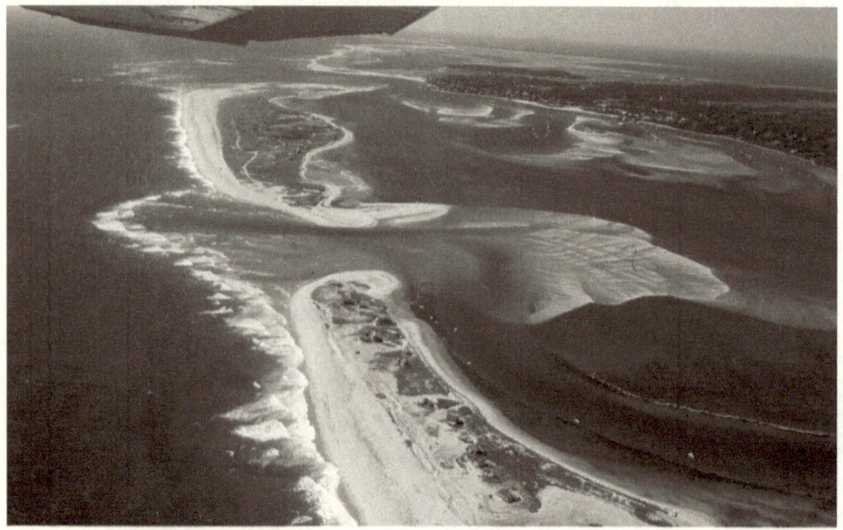

A break in Cape Cod's outer beach

Plum Island homeowners watched the February 16th tide peak at 10:56 am. It was a depressing sight. All the houses in their tightly knit community had been damaged or destroyed by the last two storms and even without storms waves were still sweeping through their Rube Goldberg seawall to undermine their homes.

But their morning papers contained even more depressing news. A consortium of federal agencies including, NOAA, NASA, EPA, USGS, FEMA and the Army Corps of Engineers had just released its most up-to-date projections of sea level rise. It made for sobering reading.

The report projected that by 2030 sea levels would rise between 10 and 12 inches on average and closer to 16 inches along the East Coast.

Coastal geologists use something called the Bruun Rule to calculate how much sea level rise will erode a coast. It is really more like a rule of thumb, but be that as it may, it states that for every foot the sea rises, the oceans will advance a hundred to three hundred feet inland. That is not particularly far but it is more than enough to wash away millions of coastal homes.

The situation is even worse if you live on a barrier beach like Plum Island. Right now barrier beach islands are able to keep up with sea level rise by rolling over themselves. For instance, after Hurricane Sandy we saw that waves had washed about 60 feet of sand off the front of barrier islands and deposited the sand in the shallow waters behind the islands. The islands were still intact, but they had migrated 60 feet inland and laid the shallow water foundation for their future migration inland.

Everything had been working fine as long as the seas were only rising a foot every hundred years as they had been for the past century. Barrier beaches could simply rollover and reform. But now that the rate of sea level rise has risen to over three feet every century, barrier beach islands will not be able to keep up. Instead of rolling over, inlets will break up the integrity of the islands and they will be entirely inundated along with any towns, villages and even cities that have been built upon them.

This will mean that states like Florida, Alabama, Louisiana and Texas will lose over 300 feet of their coasts and our only memory of places like Atlantic City will from street names on the old Monopoly boards up in our attics.

This will be will start being noticeable by 2030 and be surging along by 2050. And many communities like those on Plum Island are already spending more money on anti-erosion measures than is coming in from tax revenues.

That night, a few Plum Island residents attended a zoom session held by FEMA in nearby Rockport. Officials explained that the government had a limited amount of money to help homeowners move to higher ground. This was a hot button issue in Rockport because a number of homeowners leased land owned by the town on Long Beach. The town was considering a plan to only allow the leaseholders to remain on the beach as long as it was safe. They would have to retreat once sea level rise made it to risky to stay.

The End of Barrier Beaches

The session should have held interest for Plum Island residents as well. There were several safer lots some even on the same streets as the threatened houses. But most of the homeowners were still focused on having the city put more rocks on their seawall. But things had gone too far. The ocean had advanced halfway under and around the houses. No amount of rocks or sand would save them in the face of human missteps and the unrelenting force of nature.

CHAPTER 39
The E. O. Wilson East Coast Wildlife Corridor
Ipswich. MA

It was fitting that I was walking on Crane Beach when I heard that Pulitzer Prize winning Harvard biologist E.O. Wilson had died. He had been an inspiration when I was doing fieldwork on monkeys on Desecheo Island off Puerto Rico. Later, I met up with him in Woods Hole, in Cambridge, at New England Biolabs, and at his final home in Lexington, Massachusetts. Always interesting, interested and helpful, he wrote a blurb for one of my books that I revere to this day.

Several years ago, I bumped into Dr. Wilson with a fellow scientist at Harvard's Museum of Comparative Zoology. He asked what I was up to and I told him about my plans for a field trip to Columbia and Venezuela.

"Ah, to be 50 again," he said with his characteristic twinkle.

I had followed his work closely when he synthesized biology and human behavior in his Pulitzer Prize winning books *Sociobiology* and *On Human Nature*, but had lost track of his more recent work on the loss of biodiversity due to climate change. He had come up with the seemingly radical idea that half of the Earth should be set aside for nature.

That sounded undoable until I read his book *Half Earth*. There he explained that you could create a hemispheric habitat corridor with conservation easements and tax incentives and by building overpasses and underpasses. The path down the cordillera of mountain ranges from Canada to South America would allow nature to migrate in the face of global warming. This has already been quietly done from the Yukon to Yellowstone Park, often by many of his students now working in over 450 partner organizations like the National Park and National Wildlife services.

Suddenly it occurred to me that I was walking on a similar habitat corridor, the string of barrier beaches and barrier islands that run from New England to Florida and west to Texas. Billions of striped bass, bluefish, menhaden, herring, tuna, sharks, seals, squid and whales already use the offshore corridor and billions of shorebirds, songbirds, insects and raptors use the onshore corridor.

We are all familiar with how such species as robins, geese, cardinals, turkey vultures and even trees have moved north as the climate has warmed. Offshore species like lobsters, herring and menhaden have done the same thing. All of these species would benefit from being able to migrate to more congenial areas in the face of global warming.

But on the coasts it is the beaches and islands themselves that also need to be able to move, to keep up with sea level rise. But now many of those beaches cant move because groins, jetties, seawalls and houses anchor the beaches in place so they have no place to gracefully retreat in the face of sea level rise. The so-called anti-erosion devices only increase the rate of scour and erosion of the beaches. An East Coast wildlife corridor and conservation initiative would allow such beaches to regroup and repair themselves as they gradually retreat.

If such initiatives were extended to all the earth's coastlines the corridors of life would cover 573,000 miles, almost the exact distance from the earth to the moon.

Without such conservation initiatives, most of the world's barrier islands will be compromised and uninhabitable in 20 to 50 years at the expected rates of sea level rise. Federal, state and nonprofit conservation organizations like the Trustees of Reservations that manages Crane Beach can take the lead in insuring that residents get the legal and financial tools necessary to improve such habitat corridors in exchange for not building new houses on beaches that will be gone in 50 years.

The fitting name for this new entity would be the E.O. Wilson Coastal Wildlife Corridor.

CHAPTER 40
The Invasion
Ukraine
February 24, 2022

"Marine station, marine station. This is Russian warship.
I suggest you lay down your arms."….
…."Russian warship, go fuck yourself."
~Snake Island guard February 24, 2022

When I first started writing this book, I never thought I would have to write about nuclear warfare. It started when Russian writers noticed changes in Putin's psyche when he was isolating during the Pandemic.

As a man of action, Putin had long chafed with having to deal with long term problems like Covid-19 and climate change. Like so many people he yearned for a short-term problem he could solve with a quick thrust of brute force.

He was also haunted by festering grievances he had picked up during his days in the KGB. As an agent he had read political essays by minor Russian writers like Ivan Ilyin who expounded on the theme that the West had been constraining Russia ever since the 18th Century.

He wrote that the West (read CIA) would promote hypothetical values such as freedom in neighboring countries to Balkanize, dismember and eventually make Russia disappear.

At the same time Putin read Lev Gumilev's essays about Passionarnost, his pseudo scientific theory that Russians possess a quasi-mystical racial identity to sweep out of the steppes and conquer the decadent West … so chillingly reminiscent of the Aryan passion for lebensraum.

According to this twisted but consistent logic Putin felt that the West was now at his front door and Russia needed to strike back. It nettled that Ukraine's constitution called for NATO membership. It must have also stuck in Putin's craw that Volodymer Zelensky had replaced him as the world's new viral young folk hero while he was swiftly becoming its old reviled pariah.

If he could just replace Zelentsky with his own hand picked puppet government, Putin felt it would be the first step in returning Russia to its former glory. Russians themselves, however, were enjoying the new social and economic gains they had achieved since the break up of the Soviet Union.

At the same time, Putin knew that the United States and NATO would be constrained by nuclear deterrence. No country would dare interfere directly for fear that Russia would retaliate with its nuclear weapons.

So ten days into the invasion the world had seen the charismatic leadership of Voldomyr Zelensky and the bravery of the Ukrainian people. It had watched heart-wrenching videos of families trudging toward distant borders and the heart-warming story of a zookeeper who moved his family into the Kyiv zoo so he could sleep beside the sensitive Asian elephant Horace. When Horace woke up agitated by missiles and sirens his trainer would stroke him kindly and feed him melons until he fell back to sleep.

But the two great mysteries were the 40-mile long convey miraculously stalled outside Kyiv and Putin's ultimate nuclear plans. Apparently Ukrainian forces had stopped the convoy by disabling the leading vehicles and destroying bridges the Russian needed to advance.

Once it had been stopped, the convoy became an inviting shooting gallery. Ukrainian forces dug trenches on either side of the convoy and used javelin missiles and Turkish drones to destroy the soft easy fuel truck targets while leaving the military supply trucks for later.

But the invasion's other great mystery was Putin nuclear intentions. His first target had been the Chernobyl nuclear facility that housed 220 tons of radioactive waste and had to be constantly cooled with water to avoid another nuclear disaster. Why did Russia want to take on that particular headache?

He had also captured Zaporizhzhia, Europe's largest nuclear power plant before he had even captured any cities. Was this because they were simply

THE INVASION

easier to capture or that Putin had ulterior reasons for capturing them. He now owned two massive uncontrollable weapons of mass destruction that were being maintained by Ukrainian workers cutoff from the outside world and held at gunpoint by their Russian invaders.

Could there possibly be a more precarious situation? It was like watching an inevitable disaster unfold. Nobody had even thought about how to secure a nuclear plant in the event of a war or invasion.

Putin was using the two plants to create terror in the minds of the world but particularly in the minds of the small cadre of international workers who had spent so much time securing the facilities after the breakup of the Soviet Union. Putin had brought us to the brink of a nuclear holocaust and the world had to figure out a way to stop him so it could return to the boring old details of how to deal with climate change and our hopefully dwindling pandemic.

Chapter 41
Weapons the World Thought Would Never be Used
March 13, 2022

On the same day Russia invaded Ukraine it released documents that purported to show that Ukraine's Ministry of Health had started to destroy its bio-agents in laboratories funded by the United States.

The United States stated that this was a false flag pretext that Russia could use to justify its own use of chemical and biological weapons.

The WHO countered both countries by saying it had advised Ukraine to destroy all the high threat pathogens in its "public health laboratories" to prevent "any potential spills".

All this was all very confusing because it was clear nobody was telling the whole truth.

In fact one of the labs that Russia intended to capture had allegedly been one of the former Soviet Union's biological weapons facilities that studied anthrax. Anthrax is a naturally occurring cattle disease but in its encysted form can also be aerosolized and used a biological weapon. So the same lab could have been doing both research to prevent anthrax as well as research to make anthrax weapons.

When the Soviet Union collapsed the U.S. stepped in to provide salaries and funding to keep the Kyiv facilities in operation so they would not sell their weapons and expertise to rogue nations or terrorist groups. This was through the Biological Threat Reduction Program.

In the former days, the Soviet labs had been doing biological research similar to what was being done in this country at Fort Detrick in Maryland, the Rocky Mountain lab in Montana and the Plum Island Animal Disease Research Facility in Long Island Sound. It has also been done in government and military laboratories in Wuhan and in the Level 4 Biocontainment laboratory at Boston University.

Scientists in the labs use techniques like Gain of Function Research to identify pathogens, amplify them and discover the tick and insect vectors that can deliver the biological agents. The U.S. even has a patent to use a drone to deliver gene-altered mosquitoes over wide areas. Researchers plan to use it this summer in the United States

All this was being done under the rubric of defensive biological warfare research because its purpose is to come up with a catalogue of pathogens and their vectors so scientists could develop vaccines in case an enemy used the pathogens as offensive weapons.

However, many of these labs were what are called dual use facilities, because they were involved with both offensive and defensive biological warfare research. So while scientists on one side of the lab were carefully sequencing potential pathogens so they could develop vaccines, scientists on the other side of the lab were using the sequences to make biological weapons.

While it is now illegal to conduct offensive biological weapons research under the international Biological Weapons Convention, biological weapons continue to pop up usually when a country perceives it is losing a war only using its conventional weapons.

So it is worrisome that even before Russia captured any cities it rushed in to capture two nuclear facilities and intended to capture the Kyiv labs.

American and Ukrainian scientists associated with three of the Kyiv labs had written papers on the historical outbreaks of anthrax from 1913 to 2012. The implications of their work was that if a country uses anthrax as a biological weapon, it can make the argument that it was actually just a natural outbreak of this zoonotic disease.

One way to look at the situation was that Russia wants to put its own engineers in charge of securing the facilities. If so, we can only hope that its engineers prove to be more competent than its military commanders.

The other way of looking at the situation is that Russia will soon have three extremely dirty weapons of mass destruction. They will not be very good weapons of mass destruction because they can do as much damage to Russia as to Ukraine, Poland and other NATO countries. However, they are certainly being effective at terrifying our planet's human population.

CHAPTER 42
The Budapest Memorandum
March 22, 2022

Russia breached the Budapest Memorandum when it invaded Ukraine. If you think NATO should use that as a pretext for a no-fly zone you may be elated. If you think we are even closer to a nuclear war than we were during the Cuban Missile Crisis then you are probably relieved that the West decided to ignore the violation.

Let's look at the situation more closely. Putin has put his nuclear forces on high alert. He has used hypersonic missiles and he has intimated he will use chemical, biological and tactical nuclear weapons because he claims the West is preparing to use them.

The first thing Putin did upon invading Ukraine was to capture Chernobyl and Zaporizhzia, the largest nuclear plant in Europe. If the power were lost in either of these facilities it would lead to the release of a cloud of radioactivity that would spread across Eastern Europe. This would poison thousands of people but these numbers would pale if nuclear devices were launched either intentionally or by accident. Then we are potentially talking about the number of people killed in Hiroshima or Nagasaki.

If you think we are that close to World War III then you probably think it is fortunate the West has so far decided to ignore the Budapest memorandum.

The memorandum was promulgated after the breakup of the Soviet Union. At that time Ukraine was the third largest nuclear power in the world. Only Russia and the United States had more nuclear weapons.

But Ukraine agreed to give up its arsenal in exchange for assurance that the United States, Russia and Great Britain would come to its defense if the memorandum were violated.

While both the United States and Great Britain offered weapons and training after Russia seized Crimea, so far they have ruled out any direct intervention to avoid a potential nuclear exchange. That will become increasingly likely the longer the war drags on and the more Putin feels humiliated by his army's failings and weakened by the West's sanctions.

We can only hope that we will emerge from this war with an appreciation of how close we came to nuclear Armageddon. Some would argue that if Ukraine kept its arsenal of nuclear weapons Russia would have never started this war. But following that logic every country could say it needs nuclear weapons. On the other hand if countries only had conventional weapons the war never would have started because NATO could have countered Russia's invasion as soon as it built up its forces on Ukraine's border.

Will humanity be scared enough to finally push the evil twin genies of climate change and nuclear weapons back into their bottle? Because evidently humans are not yet mature enough to handle nuclear weapons and not yet appreciative enough of life and nature to save our planet.

But I will leave the last word to Woods Hole scientist George Woodwell. Several years ago I wrote a piece about how a nuclear exchange would destroy our biosphere through creating a nuclear winter. The founder of the Woods Hole lab that bears his name said it didn't really matter. We were either going to destroy our biosphere over a few months with nuclear weapons, or over a few decades with global warming.

Bless his soul. I hope he was wrong.

CHAPTER 43
A Turning Point?
March 15, 2022

The day before President Biden flew to Brussels to offer Europe U.S. natural gas, a river of hot air raised temperatures 70 degrees above normal over Antarctica.

The following day a chunk of ice the size of Rome broke off East Antarctica's Conger glacier. When West Antarctic infamous Doomsday Glacier disintegrates world's oceans are expected to rise 2.5 feet in 30 years. This would inundate hundreds of coastal cities and cause hundreds of millions of people to flee their homes.

But this ominous sign of climate change was barely noticed because the world was so fixated on the Ukrainian Invasion, to say nothing of the coverage of Will Smith clocking Chris Rock.

Meanwhile the world started to realize that Ukraine could actually win this almost Biblical war. Analysts were saying that Russia's 150,000 troops were not enough to both capture and hold Ukraine's major cities. They pointed out that 15,000 troops had already been killed in less than a month, which was more than had been killed in Afghanistan in 10 years. It was not lost on anyone that those losses had led to the collapse of the Soviet Union.

If you factored in the captured and wounded, Russia had lost close to 40% of their troops and the remainder were hungry, exhausted and so demoralized that the driver of one Russian tank ran over his own general, one of the seven Russian generals killed in the war. Many of the generals had been killed by young hacker drone pilots who had learned how to target and kill grey haired Russian generals. Talk about David and Goliath.

A culminating moment came when the world saw smoke billowing out of a Russian Landing craft Ukraine had attacked and destroyed in the Black Sea.

I was surprised to find myself cheering on every drone strike and counter offensive. For the first time in my life I didn't feel ambivalent about an ongoing war. I felt like my parents generation as they intently watched the Allies progress as they recaptured country after country from Hitler's grasp.

At the end of his European trip President Biden gave an impassioned speech that closed with the phrase, "For God's sake, this man cannot remain in power."

A Russian spokesman said it was up to the Russian people to decide who would lead their country and the White House claimed that it had been an add-libbed statement. But could Biden's advisers have used the President's penchant for making gaffes as a deniable cover for a well thought out message to Putin's inner circle? The Nixon administration had used a similar strategy when they publicized Kissinger's late night dates as a cover to fly him to Paris to negotiate with North Vietnam.

It seemed less than coincidental that the day after Biden's talk, Russia indicated it would stop bombing Kyiv and start negotiating a ceasefire. It made one suspicious that the U.S. might have had a mole in Putin's inner circle whose members were thinking the same thing that Biden was saying on the world stage.

At any rate, for the time being, it looked like the world might be able to narrowly escape the use of nuclear and chemical weapons and that we could turn back to facing the existential threat facing all the nations on earth.

CHAPTER 44
The Exposure
Chernobyl
April 1, 2022

"This damn war! This damn war!"

"Dymitri don't sing that. You'll have us all sent to Siberia."

"Better than this Godforsaken place. Where is this place anyway? Who ever heard of red trees?"

"Slava says it is because we're so near Chernobyl."

"This damn war!"

"You mean this military operation!"

"Yeah. Kaputin's military operation."

"Quiet here come the lieutenant."

"Quit your grumbling and dig this trench we need to have it finished before tonight. Be glad you're not at the front." (Lieutenant leaves.)

"If we're not on the front why do we have to dig these damn trenches anyway?"

"Because you never know where these Ukrainians will show up."

"Wily bastards I heard that they flew two helicopters into Belgorod and blew up a fuel depot. Nobody touched them. Where was our air force?"

"That will slow down the troops going into Donbas."

"I half hope they win this war. Next time I see a general I'm going to frag him."

"Good God Dymitri, don't say such things!"

That night Uri, Slava and Dymitri were gripped with nausea, vomiting and diarrhea. Word spread quickly through the battalion that it was because they had been ordered to dig a trench through a hotspot of nuclear waste. Everyone panicked; they had probably received a full body dose of radiation.

The following morning the battalion was transported to a special medical facility in Belarus that specialized in treating acute radiation disease.

Ukrainian officials disclosed that some of the Russian Special Forces had removed laboratory equipment and enough nuclear waste to make a dirty bomb. Was that the reason Russia had captured Chernobyl in the first place, to prevent Ukraine from building its own dirty bomb?

Would Putin use the Ukrainian pilots daring flight into Russian airspace as a pretext to use tactical nuclear weapons? Would the West feel obligated to respond? Would cooler heads in the Kremlin be able to thwart Putin's wrath? It was clear that things were coming to a head but that Uri, Slava and Dymitri would never get to see how it would all turn out.

SOURCES

Prologue

Gertcyk, Olga. *Waves of Vandalism to Mammoth Graveyards in Arctic.* The Arctic TV Chanel Yamal Region, January 25, 2017.

Patel, Kasho. *Arctic temperatures soar to an unprecedented 100 degreesin 2020.* Washington Post, 2021

Callaway, Ewan. *Heavily mutated omicron variant pits scientists on alert.* Nature, Nov 25, 2021.

Overburg, Paul. *Covid-19 drives US population to record low.* Wall Street Journal, Dec 21, 2021.

Chapter 1

It was a Dark and Stormy Night

Fountain, Henry. *North America has its hottest June on record.* NY Times, July 7, 2021.

Lytton British Columbia, Wikipedia.

Chapter 2

Living on the Edge; Water

Chen, Alicia. et al. *Rescues launched after record floods in central China displace 1.2 million.* Washington Post, July 21, 2021.

Watts, Jonathan. *Climate Scientists shocked by severity of floods inGermany.* The Guardian, July 16, 2021.

Chapter 3

Living on the Edge; Fire

Wigglesworth, Alex. *Northern California Wildfires Merge, ForcingMany from their Homes.* La Times. July 25, 2021.

Chapter 4

"We have met the Enemy and he is us."

Howard, Trevor. *There is a Fifth Horse of the Apocalypse and it is us.* Health Debate, Nov 5, 2020.

Milman, Oliver. *The carbon emissions of three Americans areenough to kill one person.* The Guardian, July 29, 2021.

Chapter 5

The TippingPoint

Kaplan, Sarah. *A critical ocean system may be heading for collapse dueto climate change.* Washington Post, August 5, 2021

Staudinger, Michelle. *A Quintessential Forage Fish; Understanding the crucial roleof sand launce.*
NOAA Fisheries report.

Chapter 6

Tesla

Dr. Cynthia Brown. Personal communication.

Chapter 7
Dragonflies

Guarino, Ben. *There's a Huge and Hidden Migration in North America - of Dragonflies.* Washington Post, December 21, 2018.

Chapter 8
Ida, Katrina and Infrastructure

Goldsmith, Wendi. Personal Communication, August 30, 2021.

Berkowitz, Bonnie. *How did Ida Compare to Katrina?* Washington Post, August31, 2021.

Chapter 9
Cobalt and Afghanistan

Afghanistan Factbox. *What are Afghanistan's minerals and resources?* Reuters, August 19, 2021.

Murdock, Jeff. *China muscle's in on Afghanistan's rare earth mineral Deposits, creates headache for Biden.* Washington Times, September 7, 2021.

Chapter 10
Cruising the Parker River Wildlife Refuge

Paul Azziz, personal communication. September 3, 2021

Chapter 11
Hurricane Larry; One Strange Bird

Heacox, Kim. *Rain Fell on Greenland Ice Sheet for the first time ever known.* The Guardian, Sept 13, 2021

Chinchar, Allison. *Hurricane Larry will produce Cat 1 Winds and … feet of snow.* CNN, September 10 2021.

Rogers, Dave. *High Tide threatens Plum Island Water System.* The Daily News of Newburyport. September 10, 2021.

Chapter 12
A Short Story about a Long Snake or Two.

Bill Sargent, Personal experience.

Chapter 13
"Guy Walks into a Bar;" Plankton Mammoth and Otters.

Zimmer, Carl. *A new company with a wild mission to bring back thewooly mammoth.* NY Times, September 13, 2021.

Temple, James. *Sinking seawater can sequester carbon.* Tech Review,September 11, 2021.

Chapter 14
The Crack in Cumbre Vieja

Ward, Steven. Day, Simon. *Cumbre Vieja potential collapse and tsunami atLa Palma*. Geophysical Research Letters, September 1, 2001.

Chapter 15

Horseshoe Crabs and Covid-19

George Buckley, personal communication, 2000. JohnHutchinson, personal communication 2021.

Sargent, William. *Crab Wars A Tale of Horseshoe Crabs, Bioterrorism and Human Health*. UPNE, 2021.

Chapter 16

Regular Gas $3.42

Bill Sargent Personal experience

Chapter 17

Sequestering Carbon Nature's way

Barker-Plotkin, Audrey. Personal communication

Harvard Forest,Wikipedia The Harvard Forest; What and Where it is. 1915.

Chapter 18

Sequestering Carbon, the Industrial Way

Fox, Kara. *The Energy Crisis Couldn't have come at a worse time for the climate*. CNN, Oct 9, 2021.

Santa Barbara Oil spill Wikipedia

Chapter 19

Methane; Glasgow's Key to Success?

McKenna, Phil. *Global Methane Pledge offers hope in lead up to Glasgow*. Climate News. Sept 20, 2021.

Chapter 19

Methane; Glasgow's Key to Success?

Chapter 20

Think Global, Act Local

Berwyn, Bob. *World Leaders Failed to bend Emissions curve for 30 years*. Inside Climate News, Oct 28, 2021.

Fickling, David. *Climate Arguments have Always Failed before theySucceeded*. Bloomberg News, Nov 2, 2021.

Chapter 21

Sharks and Seals; Worms and Coronaviruses

McKenzie, Debbie. *Seals and Cod Blog*, Dec 4,2002

Hildebrand, Lisa. *Can Marine mammals get coronavirus?* OSC Geospatial Ecology of marine Megafauna Lab Blog, 2021.

Chapter 22

Shark Attack

Mike Morris, Personal communication.

Chapter 23

Sequestering Carbon, One Whale at a Time.

Greenfieldboyce, Nell. *The Biggest whales can eat the equivalent of 80,00 Big Macs a Day.* All Things Considered NPR, Nov 3, 2021

Chapter 24

Building Our Way out of the Environmental Crisis; Will it work?

McKenna, Phil. *Global Methane Pledge offers hope in lead up to Glasgow.* Climate News. 9/20/2021

Chapter 25

The Healing

Jay Sargent. Personal communication.

Chapter 26

Resource Wars;Cobalt

Frankel, Todd. *The Cobalt Pipeline.* Washington Post, Sept30, 2016

Lithium and Cobalt A Tale of Two countries Mckinsey and Company, June 2018.

Chapter 27

The Glascow Fiasco

Mathiesen, Karl. *The last minute coal demand that almost sunk the Glasgow climate deal.* Politico, Nov 14, 2021.

Plumer, Brad. Friedman, Lisa *Negotiators strike a climate deal wouldlean far from limiting warming.* NYTimes, Nov 13, 2021

Chapter 28

Oysters: Acidification Threatens one of our proudest industries.

Poydras, Myles. *Going Deep into Oyster Country.* NYTimes, Dec 3, 2021.

Ipswich Shellfish Founder Papas Dies. Seafood Source staff March 7, 2008 Ipswich Mills Ipswich Historical Society, Oral History Notes.

Chapter 29

"Like A Big Bomb."

Hrinivasan, Hari. *The Whole Town is Gone.* PBS News Hour, Dec 12, 2021

Treismen, Rachel. *The Exact Link Between tornadoes and climatechange is hard to draw. Here's why.* NPR, Dec 13, 2021.

Chapter 30
Fusion; Energy's New Hope?

Zheng, William. *China Turns on its artificial sun in quest for fusion energy*. South China Morning Post, Dec 5, 2021

Chandler, David. *MIT designed project achieves major advance towardfusion energy.* MIT News, September 8, 2021.

Hiller, Jennifer. *Nuclear Fusion startup gets $1.8 Billion as investorschase star power*. WSJ Dec 1, 2021.

Chapter 31
The Pipeline

White, Steve. Carbon Capture pipelines offer climate aid; activists arewary. NTVNews January 4, 2021.

Chapter 32
Manganese Nodules;Cobalt for the Future?

Chapter 33
The Island

Leitner, Astrid. *A Dive into the Abyss*. NOAA Exploration, May 10, 2017.

Roach, Ann Bianca. *The obscure organization powering a race to mine the bottom of the sea.* Pass Blue, Nov 8, 2021.

Chapter 34
The Emergency!

Chapter 35
Aftermath

Chapter 36
Could Seals Harbor the Next Pandemic?

Chapter 37
"Do you have a problem with that ... Deer?"Covid-19 and Climate Change

Chapter 38
Covid-19 and Climate Change; The Seal and Deer Connection

Rogers, Nala Climate Change. *Not land use is driving deer north*. The Wildlife Society

Runstadler, Jonathan. Sawatzki Kaitlin. *Is Covid infecting wild animals? We're testing species from bats to seals to find out.* The Conversation. January 19, 2021. Questions and Answers: Results of Study on SARS-CoV- 2 in WhiteTailed Deer. US Department of Agriculture, Animal and Plant Inspection Service.August 2021.

Chapter 39
The E. O. Wilson East Coast Wildlife Corridor

Chapter 40
The Invasion

Chapter 41
Weapons the World Thought Would Never be Used

Chapter 42
The Budapest Memorandum

Borda, Aldo Zemmit. Ukraine war: What is the Budapest memorandum? NPR The Conversation. March 2, 2022.

Chapter 43
A Turning Point?

Borunda, Alejadra Antarctic Ic sheets are shatterin. National Geographic. March 2022.

Chapter 44
The Exposure

Henley Jon. UN nuclear watchdog to head to Chernobyl as Russians withdraw from site. The Guardian, April 1, 2022.

Guenot, Marianne. Chernobyl scientists accused looters of stealing radioactive material from labs there. Reuters, April 1,2022.